From

THE DAY I DIED

A story about life and all its possibilities

Ted Miller III
↑ is married to John's sister

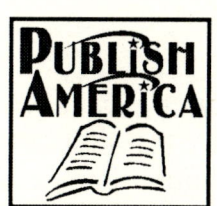

PublishAmerica
Baltimore

© 2005 by Theodore Albert Miller III.
All rights reserved. No part of this book may be reproduced, stored in a retrieval system or transmitted in any form or by any means without the prior written permission of the publishers, except by a reviewer who may quote brief passages in a review to be printed in a newspaper, magazine or journal.

First printing

At the specific preference of the author, PublishAmerica allowed this work to remain exactly as the author intended, verbatim, without editorial input.

ISBN: 1-4241-0480-7
PUBLISHED BY PUBLISHAMERICA, LLLP
www.publishamerica.com
Baltimore

Printed in the United States of America

THE DAY I DIED

A story about life and all its possibilities

Ted Miller III

CHAPTER I

    I always thought that life ended the day you died...how wrong was I.

    Even after I died, I kept on searching for a better title to this story. Because the story really isn't about death, it is about life. So please join me in this self-discovery of an everlasting existence within your own skin.

    As day turned into dark, my life receded away in shades of gray, until I was ensconced within a world where only black light existed. I knew my life hadn't always been this way. In some deep crevice of my mind I could still remember when red, blue, yellow and green ruled the visual horizons of my days. But the sense of color was fast fading away from my brain. I was trapped in a dark inward spiraling tunnel, which at its furthest end had a microscopic dot of an ever-pulsating white light drawing me minutely closer with each breath I took. During this period I discovered that death is not the opposite of life, but rather a once in a lifetime opportunity to leave a loving legacy. My passions became focused to a single pinpoint as my passage to a life everlasting was now beginning outside of time.

    My perception of pain had become but a soporific sense of soliloquy; that like the ocean's tide was high and low, but the narcotic waves of nothingness were never stilled. The wonderfully various sounds of the external world were now accented with the singular beating of my heart that reverberated and echoed in my head. With each passing moment, my self-awareness of smell and taste was less appreciated and dimmed into a dusky delusion and never more would I crave for food or drink. No longer could I detect the physical gratification of the pleasure of human touch. Not even the rain of salty tears that fell onto my face from my father's and mother's eyes could stir my voice into saying that I still loved them.

Time had ceased to exist and all of my faculties of sensation had fallen into disuse and were slowly failing at their functions. My emotions were now of the other-world that I was trapped within. In human language, this terrible trauma started out as truly an indescribable experience and was a million times worse than suffering a really bad nightmare and wondering where you were, only to discover you cannot wake up.

I wasn't living life anymore. I was one of the undead that was supported by a ventilator and surviving on electrified life support systems. Until they were unplugged, I would not be allowed to continue on my path towards paradise, purgatory or paying the penance for painful problems I might have inadvertently inflicted on other people.

The difference between my life and death became only the beeping of the multiple machines monitoring my life functions. Clear plastic tubing connected each of my body's orifices to machines that delivered or took away my vital fluids or wastes. To the outside world I was totally non-responsive, and an endless line of family or friends still could not stir my reactions with reverence or rage. My existence was now only measured by the electronic impulses indicating my internal organs were still working. I had no spontaneous movements, and my brain scans were as flat as prairie land. To everyone who passed by my bedside I would appear to be little more than a pathological vegetable. But yet deep within the dirt of the delirium I was buried, I was ever so slowly becoming calmed as my spirit was being joined as one with all I could have imagined eternity was composed of.

The prolonged period of unconsciousness I was locked within was technically an irreversible coma. I might have occasionally mimicked some conscious activities and made some sounds, but to the parade of doctors and nurses who attend me I exhibited no awareness of any external stimuli. My reactivity and perceptivity were nil. I didn't talk, gesture, have any reflexive movements or even flinch in pain when a needle would pierce my flesh. I was totally unable to react or respond to my environment. To the world I was apneic and brain dead. But deep within me and unknown to human eyes, I had a new feeling of an astral awareness that was far beyond that of my old body's functions.

In my college academic studies I learned the physical law of the universe that so states that any form of energy cannot be destroyed, only transformed into a new size or shape. For example, a waterfall turns the wheel of a turbine, which produces electricity which powers thousands of light bulbs which generates heat and rises to the sky and makes clouds condense and delivers rain to the waterfall. Energy is never lost; it is only converted into a new form.

Even though the machines of our modern world may not have been able to measure my sense of mortality, nevertheless in the neitherland I occupied, I could now understand and fully comprehend that the energy form that I used to occupy was now being changed into a more cosmic shape.

Most amazing to me was that, although I couldn't respond to any stimulus by raising a finger or opening my eyes or saying a single word in response to anything that was said, I still understood every word spoken and some that were only thought.

As the uncountable days turned into night, the feeling of my folks had changed from optimistic hope to pessimistic despair. The doctors had done everything medically possible, and now the preachers were preparing me for my earthly departure. As my family was seeking closure from my accidental death, I moved into the deepest depth of my consciousness and watched my family grant my last wish of a supreme sacrifice.

For a new beginning to an old ending, this is the time to flip the script and look up from the page you are reading. From the inside-out, see through the eyes of a dying person their last wishes.

Everyone now began to acknowledge I wouldn't complete college, go on to medical school, get married or father any children. Indeed, they now fully understood that after the machines were turned off, I would soon be in a coffin.

My dad was as pragmatic of a doctor as his father had been and knew that death and taxes were the only two inescapable and inevitable duties during life. And as such, both were well planned and provided for. We were a socially conscious family. We tithed at the church of our choice and paid our fair percentage of taxes to the government that was due to preserve democracy. We gave what money we could afford to charity and our time to good causes. We even tried to unselfishly give meaningful gifts to each other. My family wasn't super rich and not dirt poor, but we worked hard enough to know the difference between the two.

Being raised as a child of a medical doctor had its benefits and encumbrances. Education and good manners were mandatory, as well as increased social and political obligations that transcended color or creed. We were raised to know that the almighty dollar wouldn't gain you enough credit to enter heaven because it was true that some things cash couldn't buy. Although money talks loud in America, we were taught that you couldn't bid for your place in paradise. So my entire family has the ultimate final gift that would keep on giving. We had decided each of us would enable someone else to live a useful life by volunteering at our deaths to give to others our organs that could be transplanted to people who needed them.

Today, over 75,000 people in the USA were waiting for these most precious gifts, and I knew that only 5,500 donated organs had been transplanted by surgeons last year. I couldn't begin to explain what was happening to my emotions as other doctors came to examine me and later on as unknown faces of future recipients of my organs came to my side to offer my family their thoughtful prayers of gratitude. I gained a sense of peace after my mother and father put our family's donor plan into action and signed all of the final legal documents. The United Network for Organ Sharing was already aware of my situation and blood type and had matched ten organs and tissues I could donate to critically ill patients. These chosen ten had been patiently awaiting transplantation and were praying daily not to be one of the more than 10,000 people who annually die while waiting for a life saving organ to be donated.

I wanted to dare to be great and become a hero who would give the ultimate gift of life. As I finished each page of this book, I knew death could be defeated with my deed. We all know that no one's flesh lives forever. But do you realize that hundreds of people will die due to the lack of organ donations during the time it takes to read this book?

From the dark corner of my mind I gained a new sense of hope as I watched the doctors and patients discuss the parts that could be separated from my body once I was declared "clinically dead". I was in awe as I heard that my kidney, pancreas, liver, stomach, intestines, heart, lungs, bone marrow, skin grafts and eyes would all be removed immediately or within 24 hours of my death without any visible disfigurement. The doctors assured my parents that there would still be a good-looking corpse in my coffin, although they didn't phrase it that way. Even though I had lost all of my young body's sensations, I still had my sense of vanity and humor intact.

As my spirit and soul were separating from my mentality and meat, I merged my feelings into a new sponge of strange sensations and gained an instantaneous encyclopedic knowledge of almost everything. I divorced the drama of the doctors' duties and recipients' emotions and became fascinated with my body being recycled into ten other individuals. I didn't know right then what I know now was really happening to me, but somehow almost instinctively I did feel that I would still be a survivor of the chaos that surrounded my dying.

Even more amazing is that my eventual death would, in the upcoming era of time, tell of the trials and tribulations of the ten parts of my body which would be parceled out to the other people. Whether these recipients would know of or desire it, my individual sense of self being would also be merged with theirs. Our lives would prove to be conjoined for as long as they lived, or perhaps even forever more than the living human mentality can imagine. Certainly, a medical miracle was in the making, but also hidden from view a metamorphosis was too.

Upon my death and when my last wish, will and testimony would be granted, I will next enter the twilight zone which lies between destiny and dying and feels as interconnected as water and wet.

From that state of grace I will be reborn into the willing recipients and then revelations will be brought forth as my body and blood will provide an everlasting gift to all ten of us. I know this narrative might be hard to believe. But after all, where facts and figures end, faith begins.

But...I am getting ahead of those stories because I still have 28 more days to live before the day I die and start to share in the lives of others.

CHAPTER II

You already know that in 28 days I will be dead. The mirror of my mind no longer reflected the reality that most people face. During this month of mourning, the sum of all of the emotions I will experience will be so greatly exceeded that I will come to know that I am no longer of this world.

No one ever expected me to return to the land of which I was born, much less tell the tale of my death and rebirth. So bear with me while I try to defy logic and make my afterlife experience sound of human tones and tremolo. Although, it is most difficult trying to translate transcendentalism into everyday talk without sounding tiresomely techno trivial or like a blathering idiot full of pretentious theosophical trepidation.

But, it just dawned on me that you just might want to know how I got into this hospital bed in the first place.

I never expected to die young, nor did I have any predictions about the plight I was within. Like most teenage college students, I thought I would live forever.

I enjoyed the life I led. I had finished my freshman college year in good standing, and now I was gladly suffering through my sophomore year of pre-med studies.

My dad and his dad were both doctors, and it was preordained that, as the only son, I too would become a physician. It was more as if since when I was a young child, I knew there wasn't really any other occupational options that would make them proud of me. My family values had been well instilled within my moral fabric, and my parents' approval meant a lot to me.

We had lived in the same small beach town all of our lives, and my dad's and grandfather's practice had grown and thrived over the decades. We all went to church each Sunday, and I attended choir practice on Wednesday night while the family men went to the lodge. My mother was president of the P.T.A., and part-time she coached the cheerleader squad. Grandma always cooked Sunday dinner, and my sisters and I helped out doing the dishes and then we played cards. I don't want to sound like we were the perfect family living in the perfect town, but we were far removed from any inner city ghettos or gang land slayings. It was really nice to grow up safe and secure and know that your family was always there to help you with any perceived or fantasized problems.

So I never really hit that brick wall of adolescent rebellion, other than some under-age beer drinking and teenage romances that drove me out of my skin. Twice in high school I had been elected captain of the swimming team and sort of expected the same honor next year at my college. This year I again made the all-state swim team, and next year I hoped for all-American status in the 400 individual medley. Year round I swam miles of laps morning, noon and night that had helped me earn my swimming scholarship. Although my family didn't seem to need any financial assistance to put me through the university, the reward was greater than money. I enjoyed being one of the chosen few to live in the jocks' dorm within the walls of the football stadium and eat my favorite pasta meals and other dishes at the training tables along with my fellow athletes that were also loading up on carbohydrates. I was tall, tan, and taught not to be too conceited which appealed to most of the college girls I met. All in all, life was great.

When spring break arrived, I was looking forward to going back home to the beach and devouring my grandmother's manicotti and lasagna. I planned to visit with my friends who were also away at other colleges, as well as my beach buddies who were mainly slackers and sex starved surfers who couldn't imagine giving up the ocean waves to go on to more schooling. Their unspoken motto was that life was too short to not enjoy riding the surf each day. They wore wetsuits during the winter and tans all year long. I had been raised to believe that their thoughts about living life were a simplistic and silly sense of existence. But after my freak accident, I often wondered if they weren't right to master and rule the waves instead of being ruled by some schoolmaster.

Spring break went really great as friends dropped by day and night and my family fed us all. Romance was in the air, and the waves were shoulder high and rolling in regularly with high tide. Every twelve hours we would go to the sea to enjoy the blond beach beauties or sneak a beer into our bellies. Everything was good until the last day before I was scheduled to return to school. That was the day I met my future fate.

I went out early while the ocean was at low tide and flat and calm. Today I just wanted to swim some instead of surf. You could see to the cloudless horizon, and the early spring's sun touched your skin with a sense of warmth that had been missing all winter long. I set out swimming parallel to the shoreline towards the fishing pier that was about a mile away.

I swam alone because swimming is really a solitary sport. Besides that, no one I knew could have kept up with me anyways. I had been swimming competitively since grade school and should have grown gills from all of the time I spent in the water. My long, lean body sliced through the sea as easily as walking on the beach. I normally swam in indoor chlorined pools, so I really enjoyed the salt water's buoyancy and the fresh air feeding my lungs the energy to survive the pace I set. I alternated my swimming styles through the individual medleys routine of butterfly, backstroke, breaststroke and freestyle and for fun even swam some corkscrew strokes with a side scissoring leg kick.

I was only in head deep water about a hundred feet offshore. Normally I wore a skin tight Speedo swimsuit while training and slipped into a pair of baggy Hawaiian swim trunks while on shore or under the roof of our natatorium. I wasn't really modest of my body, but I didn't feel I needed to show off the size of my manhood to everyone. But today I had just worn my knee length baggy surfer shorts, and after about ten minutes I felt the drawstring loosening up. So I stopped and treaded water while I retied the knot at my waist.

I noticed a school of small silver fish race to the water's surface and jump into the air as if they wanted to fly. Then I felt a sharp tugging sensation on my right foot. It was as if an iron clamp had sprung shut and caught my leg within its steel tooth grasp. Before I knew what was happening, I was next pulled beneath the water's surface and like a wet rag twisted about back and forth. I felt as if I was nothing more than a washrag being rung out. My leg felt as if it was within a cold clamp, and the air in my lungs exploded out of me as I let loose a scream that could be heard by no one except the fish in the sea. My mind next registered a searing, raging pain that overtook all of my other thoughts, and then just a moment from passing out the thrashing movement stopped, and I fought my way back to the ocean's surface. My lungs greedily sucked in gallons of air and yet I had no energy to yell out in pain. Although my eyes saw everything, my mind was empty of any thoughts except to escape from the painful situation.

I launched myself towards the beach and tried to swim faster than I had ever done before. My right leg had grown numb and cold and my kicking was erratic and off centered. I didn't bother to pause and surmise why. I just redoubled my effort and dug deep into the water with my arm strokes to propel me towards the shore. All I wanted to do was reach the beach and run onto the sand to flee from whatever had attacked me. I furiously stroked through the waves until my fingertips touched the bottom, and then I stood to run out of the surf and towards the safety of the sandy beach. I used my arms to push my shoulders and upper torso out of the water to start my race to the shore. I took one step and with the next, fell face first back down into the knee-deep water. I stood up again and started to take another step towards safety only to fall again. People on the beach were yelling and moving towards me, but my ears didn't hear anything but an incredible loud buzzing in my head. It felt as if the blood in my brain was boiling and evaporating out of my skull and steaming into the sky.

Using my hands and arms, I crawled and dragged myself to the edge of the ocean's reach and tumbled face first into the sand. As I raised my head, the coarseness of the crushed shell-filled sand that cut into my skin was replaced with the sheer terror I saw in the faces of everyone who was staring at me. I rolled over onto my back and sat up to escape their eyes and stared back at the sea. It was then that I saw the red stain of blood in the water that I had left trailing behind me.

I was growing cold and my vision was becoming blurred and fuzzy. I could barely hear over the buzzing in my ears of the crowd shouting hysterically at each other as to what they should be doing. Everyone's eyes were wide in wonder and anyone's mouth that wasn't moving, hung wide open in an abated disgust from the grisly sight from which they couldn't turn their faces. Several women now started fainting, and one guy was wrenching his breakfast out of his stomach and onto the sand.

I started to stare at nothing except the sky as a wet suffocating smell assaulted my senses and caused my lungs to cry out for more air. Pain next started to penetrate every pore of my body. Then my mind started to go mad from the crowd's chaos. I sat still like a stone pyramid and used my arms and hands to each side of me to support my chest and head instead of toppling sideways back into the seashells and sand. I was becoming more woozy and weak, and I knew for sure I would pass out soon. I summoned what little strength I still had remaining and used it to refocus my eyes. My vision slowly moved from the horizon of the sky to the edge of the sea. The redness of the water was still growing brighter with each beat of my heart, and now even the sand was being turned sunset red.

The last real thought I would ever have in this world was not of my family, friends or even a flashback of all that I had been during the short life I lived. My last thought I had was when my eyes looked at where the trail of blood was spewing forth from and I wondered…where was my foot?

CHAPTER III

That night I felt as if I was surrounded by a ghost in the air that I couldn't touch or talk to. After I passed out on the beach, I had no memory of the paramedics tying a tourniquet below my knee or being packed in ice while, with sirens and lights paving a path through the traffic, we raced to the hospital's trauma center. On the way to the emergency room, the paramedics bagged and bottled me, using a ventilator to keep me breathing and pumping into my veins multiple plastic bottles full of intravenous fluids to maintain my blood pressure. I still had a very shallow heart beat, which was medically amazing since I had bled out five of the ten pints of blood within my circulatory system into the sea. It had gushed out of my decapitated foot like a wild river, and the decreased flow of blood led to my unconsciousness. I couldn't open my eyes, give verbal responses or move any of my muscles. You could push all of my buttons you wanted to, but no one was at home to answer your call.

The emergency team at the trauma center was waiting for my arrival at the front door as the ambulance had radioed ahead of my medical emergency. Extreme attention was directed to maintaining my respiration and circulation using intubation, ventilation, intravenous fluids, whole blood and other supportive care. They also gave me a coma cocktail, which I later learned is a mixture of thiamin, glucose and naloxone. The doctors next gave me narcotics to halt the seizures I had started to experience due to the decreased delivery of oxygenated blood to my brain. Then a renal dialysis was initiated to correct an electrolyte abnormality and to remove toxins from my kidneys while rebalancing my physiological processes.

After the trauma team felt they had me stabilized, the doctors starting checking me for severe neurological dysfunctions.

Although the hospital's personnel hoped that their actions might prompt a reversal of my medical problems, their team still started to assess my brain impairment using the Glasgow Coma Scale. They determined the seriousness of my injury in relationship to the possible outcome, and assigned my degree of dysfunction the lowest level of consciousness.

The examination assigns a different number of points in three categories involving the opening of the eyes, verbal responses and motor responses. Fifteen is the highest number of total points and three is the least possible. I scored a three! Not even a painful stimulus was sufficient to provoke any responses from me. In layman's terms, I had one foot chewed off and the other one in the grave.

During the next days the doctors administered physical exams, neurological evaluations, eye exams, metabolic blood work, urinalysis, drug screening, electroencephalographics, blood cell counts, computed tomography scans and magnetic resonance imaging. After twenty-five thousand dollars of testing, the staff informed my parents that it appeared I had suffered an irreversible severe brain injury. Although they didn't want to trivialize any medical attention, it did seem that I would remain in a persistent vegetative state of coma. Technically, I was as brain dead as a vegetable and my flat lined brain death was untreatable.

When I heard that the spectrum of my brain functions was smaller than a turnip, I thought that there ought to be a law that declares a guy who doesn't yet have to shave every day isn't allowed to die a dumb death.

During the next week, as all of my self dignity was destroyed, my awareness of information was expanded in another spectrum of consciousness and was now stimulated greater than normal intensity. Although I couldn't be aroused, my awareness was acute. In my comatose state I was in a deep state of unconsciousness, but still very much alive. I had lost all cognitive neurological functioning, but gained a higher sense of cerebral powers.

Each day I wanted to grimace or cry out that I could hear everything that was going on in my room. Each night it seemed I endured a month's worth of nightmares of believing I might remain in a vegetative state for years. It was an appalling thought of never waking up as my body would end its existence in a slow death by infection or starvation and, contrary to some medical opinions, still have full awareness despite my physical appearance otherwise.

Fourteen days after the accident the medical verdict was pronounced that my cerebrum, cerebellum and brainstem that controlled my biology of consciousness was kaput and as useless as a doorbell with no one at home.

Although my basic body functions, such as breathing, blood pressure, being awake, coordination, posture, balance, vision, and my ability to feel things, no longer transmitted my impulses through their neurotransmission system, my most complicated sensory functions of intelligence, reasoning, emotions and memory had shifted into high gear.

My level of awareness could understand my environment, even though I was apparently unresponsive and not aroused by comments or actions. My frustration at my inability to communicate was acute as my deteriorating prognosis was pronounced by the attending physicians. They declared I would always be absent of awareness and that the extent of the neurological damage I suffered would cause me to always remain in a vegetative state. Their opinion was that pneumonia would probably cause my eventual death if the tubes and wires of the life support systems remained attached to me. They further stated that only 15% of patients who remain in a coma for more than a few hours make a good recovery, and adults who remain in a coma for a month have almost no chance to regain a regular functioning life. Last and not least said was that patients whose comas are caused by massive bleed outs of the brain almost never recover. Although with continuous medical support I could remain in a persistent vegetative state for decades while the staff would focus on preventing seeping bed sores and fighting off infections and pneumonia. My coma represented the last and lowest level of my body prior to death. Finally, it was explained to my folks that, if I survived the first 28 days of observation, my decades of existence was a subject of debate that only the family could decide.

My dad was a doctor and didn't need to be told all of this. I was sure that my mom would have rather not known all of the gory details of my possible existence of when the only difference between my life and death would be the beeping of the life support machines monitoring my functioning while tubes connected to me would deliver enough oxygen, drugs, and nutriments to try to keep me from wasting away.

During heart rendering bedside talks with me, my parents searched for the answers to the problems we faced. In the end, they decided to wait out the month of observation and then have the hospital pull the plug on my physical existence.

I knew that my father in his work had faced other life and death decision, and I had witness him at home in despair after losing patients to death. But the anguish and tears he now vented were as if a volcano of feeling had erupted. Both of my parents cried a river of tears until no more could fall from their faces because of the predictable loss of their only son's life.

Next the countdown began. The proper donor agencies and social services were contacted, and then the monotony of nothingness took over the days and nights of waiting, worrying, and wondering and wishing for a miracle of science or faith to break through the barrier I was trapped deep within.

My family had been informed that there had been other long-term coma patients who when returned to the land of the living had informed their doctors that, although it appeared they had been totally non-responsive, in actuality the patients had heard every word spoken to them.

So instead of just staring at me and offering prayers to the Almighty that I may not be in pain, my family and friends talked of the news or read to me of world's events or played cards to pass the time away. My sisters even smuggled into the hospital our old family dog, Benji, who excitedly jumped up on the bed to smell my face and licked my hands to gain a final taste of my skin. I had always believed that Benji liked me best, but he couldn't stay long because he would growl and bark at anyone who wasn't in our family. Even when friends came to the house, we would have to put him in the backyard because he was so protective.

Night and day the T.V. was left on all of the time to insure that if I had to be left alone, at least I would have a little electronic entertainment. As the rest of my senses grew dim, my hearing became more attuned and acute. The story of my accident was once retold on network T.V., and I swore that my ears perked up to a point when I heard the story of how a shark had bitten off my foot. At the end of the news report, I prayed that the shark that chewed off and swallowed my lower leg had chocked to death on it, or at least contracted a severe case of indigestion.

You gotta remember that just because you are losing your life doesn't mean that you lose your sense of vengeance or humor. After all, it did seem ironic for a state champion swimmer to be out swum and sank by a shark at sea.

But the newscasters were putting a different spin on this story because shark bites were bad publicity for tourism and could cripple the local economy. So the storyline concentrated on how a doctor's son's despairing death would result in someone else continuing to live due to my organ donations. The yin and yang of my dying was showing my helplessness being balanced by the happiness of the future recipients of my last gift.

Even now I had an inkling that the destiny of my days would extend beyond death, but the depth of the dogma of my fore-coming days I could not begin to comprehend.

Being in a coma is not the most socially active way to live out your last days on earth, but at least God has granted you the time for classmates, family and friends to pay their last respects. As an endless stream of visitors passed by my bed, none of them could really be sure that I was still really here in spirit and soul. They all told me of how sorry they were as their crying stained the crisp white sheets. As their salty tears flowed from their eyes onto my cheeks, I wished I could have spoken back to them and let them all know I appreciated all that they felt. But that option wasn't in the house of cards I was playing within.

So I just played the hand I was given and didn't complain to anyone about the raw deal I was dealt. My life's luck had changed from my winning at the Friday night card games to now learning how to play solitary. I had a poker face on to all, and no one could have guessed what cards I had closest to my chest. Although I don't know how much attention my friends were really paying to our card game because I think I even won some of the poker hands we all played during my last weeks of dying a slow death.

It was during this time when I tried to figure out what cards the others were holding that I realized that God had a plan for me that I couldn't see. I came to know that every day above ground was a good day, and that the great and glorious days wouldn't start until after I cashed in my chips and was buried in a grave.

Only in your mind's eye can you imagine a life without lies or illusions. I knew that soon I would enter that world of wonderment.

CHAPTER IV

The day I died was really a relief for me. I had grown tired of being stuck between life and death and was anxious to discover what type of game I would next be dealt.

But again I am getting ahead of the story. The final two weeks of my life were a blur as a beehive of busy bodies surrounded my bed. My father had taught me to never be less than what I could be, so I learned never to follow and instead always led the way. So after pushing my short life to the limits while I was alive, would you expect me to do any less in my death?

My dad was a prominent physician in our small community and served in many social and civil positions. So the news of my accident and pending death was widely reported in local and state newspapers and eventually made nationwide coverage. The reporters who wrote the story lines were not calloused or cruel, but tried to honestly portray my family's grief being balanced by the precious gift of life my death would give to another person now dying. By the giving of parts of my body, I would enable ten other people to live a fuller and longer life.

So as a living tribute to my death, my family allowed the press to publish a series of articles about our choice to donate my usable organs and tissues. It was our hope to not only save ten people who were dying of a disease, but to also encourage other families to volunteer their organs to provide transplantations to the thousands of terminally ill patients.

Because my father was a board member of the United Network for Organ Sharing, which administered the National Organ Procurement Program, he helped our local reporters gather all of the information needed to make their articles ring with authority. His reliable links to resources and suggestions were well received by the media, and I was proud of his professionalism despite the fact that his son was dying.

The series of articles were mainly composed in my hospital room during the dead of night. After my father had attended to his patients that he couldn't refer to another physician, he came to the hospital and ate a light dinner while describing his day of dogma to my mom and sisters.

When my mother would leave to go home, dad would stay and, with a clipboard on his lap, start to write the news articles which would become a testimonial to my death. At times I could hear his tears fall and stain the ink and cause running lines down the surface of the page. And other times he wrote as if his ink pen was possessed by words seeking refuge from the rage he felt within.

The reporters came late in the evening and discussed with my dad the direction the articles were taking and what they wanted to examine. They were always very polite and solicitous and spoke to me as if they could hear the unspoken responses that couldn't escape from my head. The writers planned a most ambitious project which would not only educate and raise the awareness about organ donations, but would also chronicle the last of my days and the beginning of a new life for those who were saved by receiving my final gifts.

Of course, anyone who knew my dad would know that he wouldn't have allowed them to do anything less than their absolute best. No matter what the subject was, it had to be superior or he would shove it into the trash. So each night I listened to him patiently explaining to the reporters the medical terms into layman's language, and I learned more about organ and tissue transplants than most aspiring doctors who were still in their college school rooms.

The article would start out by answering some of the most common questions about organ donations. The first story started out by asking the question, "Would you let someone die if you could save them?" With almost a religious fever the writers went on to explain that everyone could be a hero and help end the frustrating, countless hours of an ill person awaiting their death if a suitable implant couldn't be found.

Every one of us is a potential organ or tissue donor regardless of sex or age. You don't have to be smart, quick, athletic or fit. All you've got to do is sign a donor card, make your family aware of your wishes, and at your death you become a hero. Your legacy will be heralded for your courage and celebrated for your social conscientious and generous gift of life.

To be an organ donor, brain death must occur. That means you are really dead and no longer functioning. Only after every attempt has been made to save your life, and a team of doctors who are not associated with the transplantations test and test again that all criteria to clinically declare you dead have been met, can your organ donation proceed. Hospitals also request consent from your next of kin, and if they agree, then the doctors test you to ensure you are a suitable donor without disease or infections.

Once a patient is declared dead and the family gives their consent and all the tests are completed, then the organs and tissues that may be donated include the heart, liver, kidneys, pancreas, lungs, bowel, stomach, eyes, bone marrow and skin. All of the surgery is done within 24 hours.

After the medical procedures are completed, there is no visible disfigurement to the body and an open casket is possible. Only the immediate family will know of the donations, and the law guarantees the confidentiality of the donor unless the family gives permission for the information to be released.

The debate to insure separating the dead from the dying has generated some intense discussions about the ethical propriety of removing organs from individuals whose vital functions are maintained on life support machines.

The cornerstones of this debate concern the accuracy of diagnosis and adherence to strict medical standards. The Hippocratic Oath ethic to do no harm sometimes seems in conflict with the newly developed powers in the medical arts. Recent advances in medical and surgical techniques, coupled with overly aggressive life support systems, have expanded the power of medical technology to manipulate death. In these arduous circumstances, the atmosphere is charged with complex emotions and residues of long lingering guilt for the loved ones who must live with the decision to pull the plug or postpone the inevitable demise and death of a husband, wife or child.

The legislated profile of death is an irreversible cessation of cardio respiratory activity or the absence of all brain activity. To be legally dead you are permanently unconscious with no hope of mental development, cognition or interaction with others. Some churches would preach that the cessation of all vital functions still does not mean you aren't alive because, even though you are biologically more dead than alive, you still are dying a little more with each passing day.

There will never be a clear and absolute consensus on this issue of when life ends and death begins. How parents and loved ones cope with this situation ranges from aggressive life supports to minimal, if any, intervention. We can only offer solace in these sad and futile situations and pray for the profundity of divine deliverance to the victims and their families.

However, wouldn't it be great to know that your loved one's death wasn't the final chapter in their life on earth? Some gifts money should not be able to buy, but the acute shortages of human organs available for transplanting are raising the almighty dollar's attention. Economics now seem to be gaining more emphasis than generosity. There are laws to prohibit the sale of human organs, but when money is your master, there are always attempts to dodge the directives. Organ harvesting outbids the needy population, and now the sale of skin is in the supply and demand business. Of course, these companies don't really sell organs and tissue; they just pass along a price to prepare and transport and surgically remove and then reinstall the transplanted materials. It is all very legal for these not-for-profit corporations to pay their presidents multi-million dollar salaries to procure human replacement parts, but the ethics that evolve increase the supposed myths of central American children being adopted or abducted and harvested for their body parts or a drunk and drugged tourist waking up in a bathtub packed in ice with a note informing you that a kidney of yours is now missing.

But with over 75,000 people now on the waiting list for kidneys, hearts, livers, and lungs, and U.S. surgeons only transplanting 5,500 donated organs, the law of supply and demand would warp almost any parent into purchasing a needed part for their child. You can either pay up or shut up and hope and pray that your child isn't one of the 5,000 who died last year while waiting on the long list for a transplant.

Money talks loudest in America...but it won't buy you a spot in heaven. God doesn't accept credit cards or checks. So give the unselfish gift of life that keeps on giving. Become an organ donor and place your faith in the fact that some gifts money shouldn't buy. Learn to live the dream and discover that even after death great deeds can be done.

CHAPTER V

When you die young you feel more like you are sneaking through the backdoor into heaven rather than being a saint who put temptation in its proper place and avoided the fiery rivers of hell and are now knocking at the pearly gates and asking to be let in.

As the days of my life were closing, my outlook on living changed. I began to appreciate everything for what it really was, and I was in awe of what my family and I were doing. The saving or improving of the ten people's lives that were to receive my transplants was becoming a religious experience.

Although the quality of life I was now existing was dimming, the life saving experiences I was about to gain were invigorating. I would help ten recipients to return to a normal, active life after the transplantations. Success wasn't assured, but far from experimental. One year after organ transplants, 90% of kidneys, 80% of livers, 85% of hearts and 70% of lungs will still be in excellent shape and functioning without failure.

It is said that coincidence is the intersection of where chance and fate meet. During the publishing by newspapers and national magazines of my future plans to donate my organs, a histocompatibility and immunogenic study was completed to determine the best recipients of my organs and tissues. The primary goal of the laboratory's analysis was to provide the best patients for my donations.

By examining specimens of mine, the agencies could then assess and pre-test for our cellular compatibility. These laboratories are accredited by the CAP, AABB, and ASMI to maintain the highest standards of reliability and quality. Their UNOS computer banks match blood groups, HLA antigens, antibodies, physical size of the donor and recipient, while tracing ancestry and medical history and, thus, greatly enhancing the search for a perfect match for a patient anywhere in the country.

It is not often known when a donating patient is going to die. In my family's quest to do the right thing, our mission and vision had now been expanded beyond making a difference in ten people's lives. Our goal was to now become a saga that would inspire the majority of mankind to take this giant leap of faith and become organ donors.

The primary topic of my dad's and my one-sided discussion now became how to overcome the stigma of confidentiality and instead conduct a crusade to save lives. We believed the only way the world would become aware of the acute shortages was through massive publicity. So my dad did what he always did when he wasn't absolutely sure of an answer—he called in specialists for a second opinion. He gathered in my room a local daily news reporter, a book writer, and a television anchorman. They all arrived quickly because it was well known that I was on my death bed.

With a new sense of hope guiding our way, my father assembled a team to tell the tale of my search for true transcendentalism. They soon purposed that the theme of the story would be although pride falls…love always endures.

The local audience was well aware of my story and situation, and in the surrounding cities organ donations had risen. Statewide our cause had also increased the awareness, but we wanted to launch a national news blitz about the problem of the shortages of donors. To do this, the media men knew we had to put a face and name on the people whose lives were about to be changed for the better or saved from the grave. My family had already given permission for the publicity about my organ donation, and now this news team was going to ask all of the ten possible recipients to do the same.

I only had about a week to live, and during that week it was planned to bring all ten of the best potential recipients to my bedside to visit with me and my family, and, at my ultimate departure, the transplant surgery for them would commence here at the same hospital. It was a grandstand move, but it was felt that even God would not want us to do less than our best in this situation.

My father over excelled at everything and always tried to do his best to instill the same values in all of the family, as well as his staff. But with me now dying, his zeal and energy to promote my departure into an everlasting tribute and testimonial of the theology we embrace was becoming as sacred to him as an eleventh commandment. As if an injunction had been issued by God, our crusade to save lives became philosophical in design and would explain the ultimate purpose of the natural phenomena of death. From this day forth, the goal would be that with each death may a life be saved.

As the four of them gathered around my bed to discuss the implementation of what was now a divine vision, they decided to immediately contact the coordinator of the organ donations. Over the telephone lines they patiently explained the plan and its purpose and then proposed their proposition.

The coordinator knew my father from the board meetings of the UNOS, as well as his commitment to medical excellence, and was also very familiar with our family's situation. He spoke about the question of confidentiality and said he would tomorrow contact each of the ten recipients and personally explain the situation and the degree of our family's commitment and the goal we wish to obtain.

In the closing moments of their discussion, my father reminded the coordinating doctor that the publicity would be purely professional in nature. That the public relations and recording staff he had assembled would do their best to persuade the public to understand and regard favorably the science and to also, hopefully, expand the soul searching sense of self being to help increase organ donations. That with my death it wasn't notoriety we were seeking, but rather to improve and save the lives of misfortunate people who would otherwise die.

My father wished him Godspeed in his work and with that hung up the phone. Everyone in the room then seemed to stare into empty air as if they just now contemplated the huge task they were about to try to turn into reality.

Within my silent state of grace I wanted to yell out to them, "Way to go!" But instead I had the fleeting thought, "There go I."

CHAPTER VI

Of course, my dad was successful; he didn't know how to be otherwise. The news articles were well written, and tasteful towards my terminality and the tale of the ten who would continue on with their lives due to my last gift to humanity. The local story gained statewide appeal, and the T.V. broadcast generated national attention. Money and time were donated to fly and house the recipients to my hometown, and the hospital housed all of us in the same wing.

I am sure this task wasn't as easy as I make it sound, but from my room's perspective, everything fell right into its proper place. Our local T.V. anchorman's presentation of our plight had been picked up and syndicated by its parent channel that placed our story in the national news rotation. Our strange and wonderful saga was always placed at the end of the 30 minutes of coverage, and most of the American audience had a tear or two in their eye before they were interrupted by a commercial break. Soon all three national channels carried our story each night, and home viewer numbers continued to increase as the countdown to my death and transplantation of my organs was about to begin. Our life and death situations were indeed the ultimate reality T.V. story.

During this time the T.V. showed the recipients and their families arriving at the hospital by car, ambulance and helicopter. They all seemed to have a sad smile on their face, but I was told they also had a gleam in their eyes as they looked forward to my final gift.

Each day, while surrounded by a camera crew, they walked or were pushed in a wheelchair to my bedside where they offered thanks and prayers to me and my family and pleaded with the public to not allow my death to be in vain of my family's wishes to increase the support of organ donors.

I never thought of myself as being a hero, but I was now portrayed as one. I was proud of my family and fond of my ten newly found friends. As each of their stories unfolded, I discovered a new sense of salvation. I may die, but through them be reborn with a new sense of self-discovery.

As the countdown to my demise grew shorter, my father and family also had to endure the scoffing jeers of the holier-than-thou critics, whose self-righteous piousness about my family pulling the plug instead of allowing medical machines to manipulate and mismanage my inevitable death bordered on virtuous vindictiveness.

During this time of distress, the families and friends of the recipients rained a flood of tears upon my parents in support of their decision. They openly admitted that without my parents' guidance to show the world the right thing to do, others may falter in their faith to help their non-denominational brothers and sisters during their time of need.

After all ten of my future followers had paid their tribute in prayers and well wishes, it was decided on the 28 day after my accident that the life support machines would be turned off. Medical science had done all that it could and now it was up to the Lord as to what would be my last days on earth.

That evening my room was cleared out of cameras and reporters and recipients. Only my family and minister sat at my bedside. Although I would have thought that there were no more tears available, during the bedside service the soft cries of my grandparents, father, mother and sister were accented in teardrops.

As all of the equipment was now being turned off for the first time in a month, I didn't hear the constant beeping of the monitors. As the room lights were also turned off and replaced by candlelight, I no longer felt the incandescent light on the lids of my eyes. As the tubes were pulled out of my body, I finally started to feel released from the bondage of this earth's embrace. The sharp smell of medication was now replaced with the sweet scent of the bountiful bouquets of flowers.

I felt at rest as I heard the words of our preacher explain that just because the outer vessel of our body is broken and will decay to dust, nevertheless the essence of what was within would live forever. Just because the outer clay shell will crack and crumble, the visionary vapors within will not be destroyed. That our souls and spirits may change in shape and size, but never lose their sense of life.

I am sure he said more than that and my family offered their prayers of redemption, but I had already started to take the next journey of my existence. I entered the tunnel of everlasting light that had been awaiting my release from life. My family began to fade from focus, and I then began my new adventure into the utopia of the unknowable.

CHAPTER VII

In the end I learned that I could just turn my body off. It wasn't as much as an emotional relief as an enhancement of an ethereal existence. What had been before was almost finished, and what would be hadn't yet begun. For a moment it seemed that I was stuck in the middle with no place to go. Then I realized I needed to be present at my death before I could depart for other designations. I knew without any learning that I only needed to will myself and then I could witness anything I wished to see.

So now, armed with the wizardry of a life after death, I time traveled back into the room where I died to be present and gain personal knowledge of the events about to take place. I can testify to the truth, but I can only pray that you can accept this extraordinary evidence as a confirmation of a wonderful alter-reality.

This is the beginning and end of all things I ever knew. My life would never be the same nor that of any of the ten recipients that received the organs I donated to them.

There is no money back guarantee that when you die you will go to paradise, purgatory or become a pursuivant of pain. To some of the departed, death may mean a touch of all three and to others none of the above. I came to know that it's all about the lessons we have left to learn before largesse of the Lord becomes the laissez faire of the unliving. If it sounds confusing, it's because it is meant to be. Change is never easy, and yet...it is the only constant in our cosmos.

But that's enough about the philosophical phenomenon which became my unproven paragon. I returned to the room in which I died and, like an empirical sponge, absorbed all of the actions and emotions within. No one had expected me to die as quickly as I did. But after the equipment was turned off and the tubes pulled out of me, there just didn't seem to be any more reasons to hang around in limbo. So I took my leave quickly, and now I was residing as more of an unseeable visceral vapor visiting and viewing the vigil of my death.

All of my vital functions had ceased, and the virtual image I perceived during my visitation appeared to me as rays of refracted light, which were focused and delivered into my spirit and soul.

My father had witnessed death many times before, and as an involuntary death rattle escaped from my body, he rose and put two of his fingers over the carotid artery at my throat and then, with an old-fashioned sense of superstition and medical propriety, placed a small mirror at my mouth to ensure the last of my breath had vanished out of me and now joined the cosmic vapors of the utopia of the unknown.

He walked then to my mother's side and whispered the words she never wanted to hear. As he told her that I was gone, I then was totally surprised as he collapsed at her feet and childlike wept with his head in her lap. My sisters then joined them and together they cried the tears that other living souls should never witness.

There was no concept of time on what I now thought of as my side of reality, but after their ordeal passed, they each stood and placed a kiss on my cheeks. My mother then placed my arms crossed upon my chest and pulled the freshly changed sheet over my face as dad led my sisters into the hallway where he announced to the attending physicians that I had passed away.

With a sense of grace, the medical team waited until all of my family had left the area, and then with a sense of dedication to those who were still dying, rushed into my room and started following the procedures to verify I was truly dead.

Two teams worked very quickly in conjunction to declare that I had no brain function, nor any brain stem reflexes, and that there was no spontaneous movement and I was indeed apneic. Then a ventilator was installed to resupport my lungs so oxygen could be continued to be circulated in the organs I wanted to have transplanted. I was transferred to a gurney, packed in ice, and wheeled down the hallways to a central operating theater where the donor coordinators, whose beepers had announced we were on our way, were waiting for me.

All of the surgeons and their staff knew my name, and my blood type was imbedded in their brains. As soon as their beepers went off announcing my death, the most critical of the organ recipients were wheeled first into the adjacent operating rooms, which had been reserved to ensure that the donated organs would be successfully transplanted.

Blood samples and biopsies had already been conducted to guarantee the suitability of the transplants, and the logistics of the organ removal, retrieval and transplantation had been well rehearsed. All of the necessary equipment had been assembled, as well as the various hospital departments' personnel, including the operating rooms, anesthesia, blood bank biochemistry and pulmonary units had been placed on alert status. All of the recipients' physical examinations, blood tests, x-rays and other tests were already finished, and the admitting department made sure the information was color coded and in each of the operating rooms. My medical chart was then checked and rechecked to positively ensure that the organ donation consent and brain death declaration met all legal requirements. All of this happened before the first hour of my death passed on. Now would start the test of the surgical team's skill.

The picking order of which organ and tissue was to be removed had already been established, and different teams of doctors would rotate during the twelve hours of surgery, depending upon their medical specialty. Each of the teams had also been color coded to help avoid any confusion. It seemed sort of strange being surrounded by a rainbow of strangers instead of family and friends, but in a way it also helped me stay emotionally detached from my old body as it was being stripped for spare parts and skin. Like I said before, just because you die doesn't mean you stop being comical. After all, God must be some sort of amusing jokester, because who else would have put long necks on giraffes instead of just making all the trees shorter? Although I am sure that before you finish this book, you will wish that the surgeons would have first removed my sense of humor.

The time to start the surgery was drawing near, and all of the equipment, personnel and patients were again checked and rechecked for any irregularities. The outcome of this procedure was being followed by millions of television viewers and newspaper readers and as such no one wanted any mess ups or mistakes.

So with a military sense of precision unmatched by the pentagon, they began to divide my body into ten additional parts, and although I didn't yet know it, my sense of self being as well.

CHAPTER VIII

The first organ the surgeons dressed in red removed from me was my kidneys. So from beyond the grave, thus this new story started.

Every working hour an American dies while on the waiting list for a kidney transplant. I would save but one of them. The lucky recipient's name was Adam and both of his kidneys had failed due to pyelonephritis. The dialysis catheter hanging out of his shirt told of this life-threatening failure, which is the most common of the kidney diseases. This inflammation is caused by a bacterial infection that starts in the bladder, and then the obstruction interferes with the flow of urine. If the body's immune system becomes impaired, then glomerulonephritis may also occur. This is when antibodies and other substances become formed as large particles and are trapped in the glomeruli.

But I sense that I had better back up a little because most people don't have a clue as to what their kidneys do or even where they are located. You may have heard about getting kicked in the kidneys or a kidney bean or a kidney stone or even eating grilled kidneys for breakfast if you live in England, but their function and structure remains a mystery to most folks.

At the university during my pre-med studies I had already completed basic biology and advanced anatomy, but I still could find myself getting lost in the human body without a road map marking the meat and muscles of mankind.

During my introduction to the kidneys' structure and function, it was explained to me that the human kidneys are two fist-sized, bean-shaped organs that are reddish brown in color. They lie against the rear wall of the abdomen on each side of the spine and are situated below the middle of the back. Your liver is to the right, your spleen on the left, your stomach to the top and your bowels below.

The gross anatomy of your kidneys is divided into three regions – the outer region is the renal cortex, the renal medulla lies on the inner side, and innermost is a hollow chamber called the renal pelvis. Microscopically each kidney is composed of about one million tubules called nephrons. These tiny tubes filter your blood to remove uric acid, nitrogen-containing compounds and other wastes in the form of urine and regulate the amount of fluid in your body.

When you hear someone sarcastically say that their kidneys are about to float or burst, it means that their urinary system is over-filled and they feel a discomforting pressure or a sharp pain in their lower back which will be relieved by emptying their bladder of urine.

The way your kidneys work is blood first enters through the renal artery, which divides into smaller blood vessels called arterioles, and eventually continues to get subdivided into the tiny capillaries of the glomerulus. Once within this cup-like structure, your blood pressure is very high and the thin capillary walls allow the water and wastes to be pushed out and collected in the Bowman's capsule, which is a depository and drain. The blood's red cells and protein molecules are too big to pass through the walls, so they leave the glomerulus through another arteriole which branches into a network of blood vessels that are lined with tightly packed microvilli that act as a brush border. This passage filters and traps the waste products contained in the 50 gallons of blood that moves through your kidneys every day. But along with the wastes that are in your blood, the filtrate which has been trapped also contains water, salt and nutrients. So while these liquid wastes continue their passage to your bladder, they first pass through your renal tubule and, in an important process called "tubular reabsorption", enable your body to selectively keep 99% of the substances it needs while ridding your body of about 1.3 quarts of urine waste each day.

Your brain monitors your kidneys' functions and if too little salt, water, or other substances are in your blood, then the hypothalamus, which is located in your head, causes vasopressin to be released and the antidiuretic hormone makes the openings in the renal tubules and ducts more permeable to water. Another hormone called aldosterone, which is produced by your adrenal glands, then causes constriction which helps keep your blood's salt level and blood pressure in the best narrow range for physiological activities.

Your kidneys also adjust your body's acid-base balance to prevent the blood disorders of acidosis and alkalosis and produce several hormones, which stimulate the production and release of more red blood cells from your bone marrow.

Your kidneys are so vital for living that, like your lungs, eyes, and ears, God gave you two of them in case one might fail.

Adam hadn't been lucky. Even though he didn't drink or smoke and exercised regularly, both of his kidneys had failed, and his life was only sustained through the treatment of kidney dialysis. He didn't have a living relative to donate a kidney, and so he survived on the dialysis machine. In this procedure his blood was circulated through a machine that employs the principle of passing the blood through a semi-membranous tubing which is surrounded by salt and other small molecules saturated in a solution so that the wastes will diffuse through the membrane into the solution and the blood cells and plasma proteins stay behind and are returned to the patient. Every day he had to go through a six-hour treatment to remove approximately 250 grams of urea. Without being hooked up daily to this machine, he would die.

Even with this machine assistance, Adam still suffered symptoms of fever, chills, and back pain. He also took tons of antibiotic drugs to fight off infections which left him in a drugged dazed state for most of the time. The cost of his operation wouldn't be cheap. A kidney transplant costs $111,000, and many insurance companies will not cover the costs. But he knew that money won't do you any good after you are dead.

Days ago when he was first wheeled in to visit with me and my family, I could hear the chattering of his teeth, and my father had asked him if he needed another blanket to help against the cold he was experiencing, even though it was 90 degrees in the shade outside.

Adam and his wife spoke to my family and reporters of how

grateful they were with my gift of life and how it would change forever their lives. They knew there are almost 55,000 people on the waiting list for a kidney transplant, and the average wait is over 500 days. Annually there are less than 6,000 registrants willing to donate their kidneys, of which 5,000 are relatives giving living donations. And as such, the death rate on the waiting list is over 90%. This is the highest death rate during the last decade. Since Adam was diagnosed with this death sentence, his life consisted of not knowing or caring what day it is and only wishing and hoping against all odds just to see another new day.

This surgery isn't new. In 1954, the American surgeon, Joseph Murray, successfully transplanted a kidney donated by the recipient's twin brother. Now through the sacrifice I would make of my body, Adam would live and have a 94% successful survival rate chance.

With the camera crew recording the moment for all of prosperity, Adam stood from his wheelchair and declared with tears in his emotionally choked voice that if only I could see what he saw in his eyes, then there would be no doubt to anyone in this world that I am a hero. His family would be forever in debt to mine, and he could only pray that somehow this message would reach me. Then he collapsed and fell back into his wheelchair, and I didn't see him anymore until today.

From my floating position in the air above the operating table, I could see with a new sense of sensation through the hospital's wall and perceive Adam in the next operating room. Below me laid my body, which was now being prepped for surgery. To avoid any mistakes each surgical team, their equipment, and documentation was color coded.

This medical event was a milestone because ten surgical exchanges at one location had never before been performed. It was becoming more than a dramatic sense of survival. For future transplant recipients, this was the dogma of a new dawn as death was closing in on their days.

As the first team of doctors and their assistants all dressed in red were standing around my body, I felt a twinge of trepidation when I saw the scalpel slice through my skin. From my throat to my belly button, the surgeon followed the iodined marked lines and continued his incision to each of my hipbones, marking an upside down Y through my skin. With swift and accurate moves, the edges of my skin were next folded back and away from the incision, and forceps were clamped and attached to the skin's edge to hold it away from the inner cavity of my body.

During my years of swimming I had gone skinny dipping many a time, but never before had I felt as exposed. I knew the body I used to rule was now but a cadaver, but to see my muscles moved aside and all of my inner organs exposed was more than a wonderment to me. I could identify my entire digestive tract from my diaphragm to my intestines. As my blood was being suctioned and siphoned aside, you could make out the individual organs. Their color ranged from the pink of my stomach and small intestinal walls to the rust red of the liver and was accented by the green of my gallbladder. The surgeons hadn't yet split apart my breastbone to expose my heart and lungs because the surgical teams first wanted to remove all of the donated organs from my abdominal cavity.

The kidney transplant team was the first of the ten teams waiting that before 12 hours would pass would remove from my old body the kidneys, pancreas, liver, stomach, bowel sections, heart, lungs, bone marrow, skin, and eyes.

The kidney team of surgeons very carefully pushed aside my stomach and liver, and proceeded to first inspect both of my kidneys for any sign of distress or disease. Next they surgically loosened the surrounding tissue, taking great care not to damage the adrenal glands or gallbladder that sat in close proximity. Then the surgeons sealed off the arteries and veins as they continued to cut away the transparent fibrous membrane called the renal capsule, which helps protect your kidneys against trauma and infection. Finally they flushed the organs with a preservation solution before removing my kidneys and packing them in ice inside a red cooler.

Then as quickly as they began, they left to inform Adam and his family that the kidneys were healthy and suitable, and then immediately started his anesthesia before his surgery would begin.

As another team that would next remove my pancreas now took their spot at my table, I couldn't resist wanting to go watch my kidneys be reinserted into Adam. I didn't have far to travel because he was in the operating room next to mine. Adam was attached to a bank of monitors and machines and being attended by an army of medical workers. His dialysis catheter, which was always attached through his yellowish skin, was now joined by a host of others.

The surgeons sliced him up much less than me, and in five hours his surgery was completed. While he would be lying in the recovery room, he would notice a pinkness in his hands when he would press his palms together in prayer. He would stare at them in wonder and then realize his blood wasn't contaminated anymore. One transplant had been successful, and his family's prayers and mine had both been answered.

During Adam's and my forthcoming years of being conjoined together, I felt more alive inside of the dead zone I was within than ever before while I was still breathing. As Adam's years would go by, he and his wife had another child and named him after me. During the next decades, Adam would dream about me and what I might have been doing if I hadn't died. Some days he would feel as if my spirit was visiting with him and watching my namesake grow up from being a baby and into a young man. Adam never really saw me, but he could feel my presence in almost all he did. One of the stranger side effects was after his prayers were said and his days of labor were over, sometimes he would experience a most unusual feeling. Even though he still didn't drink any alcohol, on some Saturday nights he could taste the scent of beer on his breath and feel a little intoxicated. It was as if my memories of the nights of me attending a beer bash on my college campus were now his to enjoy as well.

Life is strange, death is stranger yet. In my new role as a guardian angel, I discovered it was as if heaven was one gigantic library and everything you could ever want to know is at your fingertips. I came to realize that this journey of our lives has a destiny beyond death. I had now reached the land where God's only rule was for you to do your best.

CHAPTER IX

My pancreas would be the next part of me to be picked out of my dead body by the blue team. Diseases of the pancreas are not common; however, Paul had been diagnosed very early on as suffering from cancer and acute pancreatitis, and this serious condition, if not relieved, would most rapidly cause his death.

Most people's problem with their pancreas is that it is not producing insulin. This condition is normally brought on by a viral infection that causes cytotoxic T cells to destroy the pancreatic islets of the Langerhans. These ill individuals must have daily injections of insulin or suffer the symptoms of hypoglycemia. This low blood sugar state can cause unconsciousness since the brain requires a constant supply of sugar. Diabetics are also prone to blindness, kidney disease, circulatory disorders and strokes.

Your pancreas has both exocrine and endocrine secretions made up of a number of enzymes that are discharged into the intestine to aid in digestion. Insulin is produced in the glandular cells of the pancreas known as the islets of Langerhans. The failure of these cells to secrete sufficient amounts of insulin causes diabetes. If untreated, the resulting buildup of ketones in the blood supply reduces your blood volume and produces acidosis. Next your acid blood can eventually lead to coma and death.

Back in 1920 the physician Banting and his lab assistant, Best, spent a summer in a University of Toronto laboratory where, due to limited funds, they worked, slept, and ate in the lab. By the end of the summer, they obtained pancreatic extracts that by 1922 were purified from pigs and cattle, and this insulin is presently synthesized using recombinant D.N.A. technology. They received the Nobel Prize for their work in 1923.

Paul knew he was lucky to get my pancreas. Most kidney patients whose organ failure was caused by diabetes mellitus also receive a pancreas transplant at the same time. Last year there were less than 450 pancreas transplants performed in the United States.

When Paul visited with my family and me, his systems were acute. The peritonitis he suffered was much worse than an intestinal obstruction. The hemorrhage of his pancreas had caused a serious, generalized infection of his abdominal lining that looked as if his appendix had burst open and spread its fluid infection throughout his intestinal tract. His belly had swollen and jaundice coated his skin and colored his eyes yellow. He looked like walking death and knew he didn't have long to survive without a transplant. As I sensed him there and heard him speak to my family, I could smell a stale, sweet stinking odor in his sweat. The glucose in his body was no longer being metabolized nor stored in his muscles or body cells as glycogen. The glycerol and fatty acids in his body were now being leached out through his skin, and my super sensitive sense of scent was detecting it in the air surrounding us. No amount of perfume or deodorant could disguise the coying smell similar to that of the skin of decaying fruit. I felt so sorry for him, and yet I could not say a word to lessen his load. I knew of his mixed emotions of not wanting to see someone die, but yet if I didn't pass on quick, then he too would soon die.

Paul was already anaesthetized and in a stupored state of sleep as his blue clothed operating team was next assembled around my table. They first inspected my pancreas and determined its size and shape was as it should be. It is a conglomerate gland that lies transversely across the posterior wall of the abdomen, which is about eight inches in length, about three inches wide and an inch thick. It only weighs about three ounces and its head lies in the duodenum cavity, which connects your stomach and small intestine. Your green-colored gallbladder sits above and to the right of your pancreas and is connected to it via a common bile and pancreatic duct.

His surgeons were well aware that our successful pancreas transplant would be notably difficult. As the doctors who were wearing the dark blue scrubs swapped our organs, they knew that the first transplants were performed in 1968 at the medical school of the University of Minnesota. And even with the advent of anti-rejection drugs such as cyclosporine, which is a natural product found in a soil fungus, only about ten percent of the pancreas which are harvested and transplanted last for more than one year. But with each suture, they could only hope that the stitch would save some time. They knew that when your life expectancy is now as Paul's, measured in hours instead of days, weeks, months and years, every single breathing moment becomes precious. Paul had been living on borrowed time for a long while. The odds of him surviving were difficult, but so had been the 30,000 to one chance that his and my histocompatibility of over 200 different antigens being acceptable to each other had properly matched up. As the surgery was drawing to a close, we both knew that our chances of surviving were long shots, but, after all, our odds were better than the chances of winning the lottery. We were well aware that if you didn't play in the game of life, then there was no chance at all of winning.

The providential discovery we wanted to seek would still remain in the horizon of each divine additional hour we breathe and eat until our final intervention occurs.

So although our odds of living a long life were slim and our confidence and hope were fast fading away, what remained for both of our spirits was an inner sense of serendipity and sereneness not achievable in normal life.

CHAPTER X

My liver was next on the list to be lifted from my body. Linda was the lady's name who would be the next to benefit from my brave bravissimo. Her family was willing to move heaven or hell to try to get her a liver transplant. Linda was only 16 and she had contracted Hepatitis C during a blood transfusion that had destroyed her liver. It happened when, during a South American church youth rally and sabbatical, she had drunk water which had been contaminated with sewage. Upon an initial attack of Hepatitis A, a blood sample of hers had been accidentally withdrawn using a contaminated syringe needle.

Her family had even been driven to consider taking on the ethical issues that are ever growing in the transplant wars. Although organs cannot be legally bought or sold in the United States, the access to good medical care still requires either an outstandingly good insurance plan or $250,000 cash. For families who are not willing to wait in the long line for a transplant while their loved one dies, some can use the power of the dollar to get a donation. They reasoned that just because other patients whose organ failure was the result of their own actions, such as trying to drink themselves to death and have caused cirrhosis of their liver from alcohol abuse and are now on their third or forth liver transplant because they are deemed a top priority in the line, is not a valid reason for their child to die. With few exceptions, the donated organs go to the person closest to death, even though their prior transplants failed and are known not to do as well as a person who has not already had a liver transplant.

Money is already a major issue because you can't even be put on the transplantation waiting list if you cannot prove you can pay for the quarter of a million dollars of surgery. So since the poor patients will die due to their lack of dollars, why shouldn't the super rich exploit the Far East black market? In China the bodies of executed prisoners provide the source for people willing to pay cash for organ transplants. Linda's parents were not rich, but were wealthy in the ways of the Lord. Their church was raising funds to help finance her surgery, and her parents and grandparents had remortgaged their homes to give their daughter a second chance at life. It was a crying shame that some contaminated water in a far away land that she drank during her service to the Lord was now taking her life. Linda was just turning 16, didn't take drugs and was now dying because of some third world medical mistake causing an unsterilized needle to transfer a virus to her body oncogenes that altered the genotype of her liver's cells, which repeatedly divided into cancerous divisions.

I knew from my previous pre-med studies that the liver has amazing regenerative power and, in some instances, can repair damage done to it and heal itself. It is also the only organ that can grow back to its original size. In many liver transplants, the organs can be obtained from a family member or friend who donates a portion of their liver to the patient and then, after the diseased section of the bad liver is replaced by grafting the good liver to it, the liver can grow back to the same size as before the operation. Also, if the liver damage is not too severe, then a temporary transplant can take over the ill liver's function while the patient's own liver recovers.

The two types of transplants can be artificial livers or xenotransplantations. The developed artificial livers consist of a cartridge that contains healthy liver cells, and your blood passes through a cellulose acetate tube and is serviced in the same manner as a normal liver while your sick liver has a chance to recover.

Although liver transplants are the preferred treatment and artificial livers have been tried in some cases, there is also a third alternative called xenotransplant. Due to the acute shortage of donors, some surgeons now use animals as donors. The animal receiving the most attention from the medical community is the pig. Surgeons in the United States transplant about 60,000 pig heart valves into human each year, and these tissues are not rejected by human bodies. However, it used to be that transplanted pig organs undergo hyper acute rejection when the recipient's immune system recognizes the organ is foreign and the blood vessels shut off the delivery of blood to the pig's liver and it dies. Nowadays scientists use genetic engineering techniques to breed pigs with the antigens found in human blood vessels. These transferred proteins and polysaccharides fool your body into not producing an antibody because of the presence of a foreign antigen within you. So now livers from these specially bred pigs have been successfully connected to the bloodstream of ill patients to clear away toxic wastes while the patients' own livers recover and regenerate on their own.

The biggest drawback of xenotransplants is that unknown and possibly deadly viruses could be transferred from the animal to mankind. And once within humans, they could be spread or bred into other humans with unpredictable results.

But neither Linda nor her family had to face this unresolved question because only in non-severe conditions can a temporary transplant take over the ill person's liver functions while it regenerates and recovers. Liver failure due to cancer cannot grow itself back healthy due to the cancer cells continuously attacking and converting any new cells. Her entire liver would have to be removed, but with the grace of God, the initial biopsies indicated that only her liver was infected.

Ever since being diagnosed, Linda and her mother had been living in the hotel that was next door to the clinic and praying to be one of the 4,900 people this year who would receive a transplant and not one of the hundreds that will die while awaiting their name to move up on the list.

But Linda was lucky because my father was familiar with her case and had developed an exception of ethics for her treatment. My dad was on the treatment staff for transplantations and as such recognized the difficulty her family faced. Linda needed a transplant or she would die. But she had to have one foot in the grave before she could move to the top of the list. So instead of her waiting to be re-evaluated and ranked and placed on a computerized waiting list, my father had instructed her family to remain in this area instead of going home. He knew when a donated organ does become available, it is first offered to patients in the donor's area to reduce the risk that the organ could be rejected due to time and travel. If no one locally can undergo the major surgery, then the organ is next offered regionally or, in rare cases, elsewhere in the United States.

Linda was undergoing daily treatment at the hospital to insure her maximum healthiness, and all of her medical records were up to date, color coded green, and now stored next door to my room with the other nine people's different colored files who would receive their transplants from me. Then to absolutely insure the proper procurement picking order, my family signed the permission forms that as a living donor I could donate my blood, a kidney, portions of my liver, and any other partial tissues or organs should I survive being disconnected from the life support systems.

This fact was never made publicly known to anyone except my family and the immediate physicians because no one wanted it to appear as if my parts were being harvested from me while I was clinically brain dead but still alive.

Medically speaking, my family knew that there was no hope in me recovering after being in a deep unresponsive coma for 28 days, but when I learned that I could just turn my body off, there was no reason for them to feel they were taking any parts from me before I had perished.

I learned a lot about Linda and the liver because she often sat by the side of my bed and, although I didn't reply, she read to me volumes of material about digestion, nutrition and the liver's functioning. She was a straight A student in school, and now it was her life's plan to become the physician that my dad had wanted me to be.

I knew Linda's symptoms had advanced from a constant state of being tired and the yellowing of her eyes and skin to severe itching, easy bruising and a tendency to bleed easy and now advancing to muscle loss and an abnormal buildup of fluid in her abdomen, accompanied by dark urine and grey-colored stools. Next she would face the vomiting of blood and mental confusion before a coma would claim her.

During our daily one-sided bedside chats, Linda explained to me that the liver is the largest organ in the body. It is located on the right side of your abdomen and rests below your diaphragm and lungs and above your stomach. It is also one of your busiest organs and performs more than 400 functions each day, including detoxifying the blood, aiding in digestion, distributes nutrients found in food, produces blood clotting and other important proteins, filters and removes any drugs or alcohol consumed, stores fats, sugars and vitamins for later use, and destroys and converts your old worn out red blood cells into bile which is then stored in your gallbladder. Your liver has so many functions that it is essential to your cardiovascular, urinary and digestive system and you cannot live without it.

Linda went on and on explaining all of the details and interaction and chemical balancing your liver functions for, as well as the disorders that affect the entire liver and hinder its ability to repair itself. Along with viral hepatitis and cirrhosis, which mainly attacks Europeans and North Americans, there is also a tropical parasitic trematode worm that causes schistosomiasis. In the Middle East, Asia, Africa and South America, millions of people are infected and die each year from these blood flukes. This extreme disease is caused by skin contact with water-borne larvae with your feet. The adult worms live and copulate in your blood vessels, and their eggs migrate into the digestive tract and pass out with feces. Then they hatch out into tiny larvae that swim in the water until they infect a snail and when its asexual reproduction occurs, new larvae forms and leaves the snail and if they penetrate human skin, these sporocysts mature in your liver and small intestinal blood vessels. Those who are infected continue to physically weaken until a secondary disease brought on by their condition kills the human host but not the worms. At the end of a week, I knew more about the liver and its possible disorders than I ever cared to know. I was glad though that Linda didn't have to get her new liver from someone who worked in a rice paddy and then perhaps have to face another whole list of problems.

Linda was already in the third operating room when my liver was surgically loosened by the green colored team and disconnected from the bile duct, surrounding arteries, and portal vein and then flushed with a preservation fluid before being finally removed and placed in cold storage within a green box.

While the donor team was procuring my liver, the recipient team who was also dressed in green was preparing Linda. After she was anesthetized, her surgery began and the diseased liver was removed and my healthy liver was put in its place and all of the ducts, arteries and veins were reattached before the tubes were pulled out of her and the skin was sewn shut again. Meanwhile, new medications were continuously delivered into her blood stream through the I.V.'s to help prevent her body from rejecting its new liver. After eight hours, the surgeons were done, but Linda's recovery would take several weeks. She then would lead a dramatically improved, healthy, normal life.

As our years together would pass by, I would get to subliminally see Linda graduate first from high school, then college and next accepted and commencing from medical school. She specialized in internal medicine. I discovered through her art of learning the passage of another life that I might have led. I also learned to stop thinking as if her liver was mine and instead accepted the fact that it was ours.

Linda never lost touch with my family because my father became her sponsor in medical school. When my grandparents and mother died, she was by my father's side, and when he also passed away and we were attending his funeral, I could feel her deep sense of remorse and sorrow.

And then, in my own grief, just as I felt a kiss escape from my lost lips that I knew was doomed to never find its desire, Linda leaned forward and placed her lips upon my father's face and gave him the kiss on his cheek that I so dearly had wished for.

CHAPTER XI

By now I can't remember when I had quit being hungry and no longer drooled at the thought of my grandmother's pesto and pasta. Even though I had lost my appetite, it is said that an army marches forward on its stomach. But after seeing mine with only my bowels to keep it company, I knew my stomach wasn't going to grow any legs and walk away.

Steve was the recipient selected to receive my stomach for experimental surgery. I can remember well when the tall, lanky adolescent boy came walking into my room. My mother gasped as Steve was introduced and later made the comment that when he turned sideways he almost disappeared. Thin as a bone, this twelve-year-old was suffering from some unknown ailment that had turned his stomach into a mass of bleeding ulcers.

When at the age of ten he began to complain that his stomach hurt all of the time, his parents initially dismissed his sickness as a normal childhood's bad belly and treated his symptoms with over-the-counter remedies as millions of parents have done during past decades. First they thought it must have been something he ate that upset his belly, and after a couple of days that maybe he had the stomach flu. When Steve's bad digestion didn't end after a week, his parents then took him to a doctor who recommended a change of diet with no spicy or acid foods and wrote him a prescription for a mild anti-nausea drug. By the end of the month Steve began spitting up blood and passing bloody stools. He was next immediately admitted into the hospital and underwent a battery of tests. Among these procedures, the doctors used an endoscope to view the inside of his stomach. This long tubular instrument with a tiny lens and light source was threaded through his mouth, pharynx, esophagus, throat, and then displayed the inside walls of Steve's stomach, which now instead of being pink and thick were worn thin and almost completely covered with bleeding ulcers. After a microscopic section of his stomach wall was removed the next day, it was determined that the thick layer of mucus that normally protects the stomach walls was missing and his entire stomach lining had been massively infected by an acid-resistant bacterium. These helicobacter pylori had attached themselves to his stomach's epithelial lining. The infected areas then became exposed to his gastric gland juices which contained so much self-produced hydrochloric acid that all of the cells that secrete mucus had been destroyed. Now the wall lining of Steve's stomach was paper thin and could massively rupture at any time.

There was no good scientific reason or medical abnormality to account for Steve's stomach destruction at such an unheard of and alarming rate. The growth wasn't cancerous, but it was spreading faster as each day went by. The disease appeared to be localized only in Steve's stomach and had not spread to any of his other internal organs. The medical decision soon reached was to remove his entire stomach and connect his esophagus directly to his duodenum and pull up part of his small intestine to make up the difference in space.

My family was growing tired of the vigil they kept, but never became impolite or rude. Most of the time it was easier to listen to someone else talk than be alone with their own thoughts. As Steve's family sat with mine, my dad asked his mother and father how and when the proposal was initially put forth to them for their approval. They answered that at first they researched and read everything they could about human digestion and nutrition.

My mother and father during the weeks of my demise had become weary of making conversation. But having nothing better to do, I just laid still in my bed and listened to these strangers spend hours discussing the stomach. They started out by explaining that humans have a tube-within-a-tube body plan that starts out with a mouth and ends with an anus.

Although I am sure my father knew all of what he was being told, he patiently listened to them. He knew that Steve's parents also had to have their say and declare their duty towards my death.

But one of the things I didn't know was that an American mid-nineteenth century doctor named William Beaumont first discovered the stomach was much more than a mere storage organ whose two liter capacity of partially digested food allowed us humans to eat relatively large meals and then be able to spend the remainder of our day on other activities. This major difference between man and beast would allow humans the time to spend on developing ourselves, instead of like omnivore and herbivore animals having to graze all day and regurgitate their cud when no longer feeding.

Dr. Beaumont had a patient named St. Martin who had been shot in the stomach and after the doctor helped heal him, the patient was left with a hole in his side. Through this accidental opening the doctor was able to look inside the stomach and watch the muscular walls contract vigorously and mix and mash up the food within with gastric juices that aided in digestion. Then he discovered the juices could be produced independently of food being in the belly and that these fluids contained hydrochloric acid. The doctor determined that the acid that was secreted by the stomach's walls was sufficiently strong to kill off bacteria and other micro-organisms found in food. Then the thick, soupy consistency called chyme exits the base of the stomach through a tube by the contracting and relaxing of the sphincter muscle.

The study of the digestive gland secretions actually began back in the late 1800's when Pavlov proved that dogs would begin to salivate at the ringing of a bell that he had trained them to recognize when calling them to eat. After months of conditioning, at the sound of the bell ringing, the dogs would start to drool even if no food was present. His experiments proved that even the mere thought of food could cause the digestive system to start the secretion of gastric fluids. Without these gastric glands, hormones and secretions, then protein and fat rich foods cannot be properly processed, digested or absorbed.

Today highly improved surgical techniques take advantage of these facts. When an obese patient who suffers a life-threatening symptom cannot lose weight by diet or exercise, surgeons can tie off the majority of their stomach cavity. With this removable knot in place, most of what is eaten just passes straight through the patient's digestive tract without any fat or protein being absorbed.

But what goes in must come out, and that was what Steve's problem was about. Because he had no stomach at all during the last two years, he had grown to be extraordinarily thin, uncoordinated, and weak. Although he could continue to survive without a stomach by living on a special diet loaded with supplements and vitamins, he would never live a regular life. With his stomach removed, he could never again eat the foods he used to enjoy and provide him energy. Gone forever was his mother's fried chicken and cheese grits and in their place he existed on regimented gruel. Because his body's metabolism was unable to assimilate normal food, he was now starting to suffer from secondary symptoms and disabilities because mutagenic agents were not being eliminated from his bowels due to the development of intestinal polyps. He also now experienced night blindness, plaque formation on his arteries, defective mineralization of his skeleton, and a reduction in his nerve conduction and muscle contraction which was causing massive coordination problems.

Steve was the best candidate for the experimental stomach transplantation which just might change this sickened teenage boy into a healthy human being again. The cost of this new procedure would not be covered by any insurance company or governmental agency because it was considered experimental. But the intensive media campaign that had been locally organized was starting to take hold of the hearts of Americans and had loosened the hold of those who held the public purse strings. A private foundation agreed to fund the expenses of the transplantation and a team of university doctors agreed to work for free.

At the end of our families' session, when all that could be said had been said and the tears of gratitude and grief had dried, Steve had one last question for my dad. He said he felt sort of stupid but had to ask if there would be any influences or problems about our compatibility since he was black and I was white. In his best bedside manner, my dad medically explained to the twelve-year-old that it was our blood type and other histocompatic antigens match that were important and not our race or families' histories.

THE DAY I DIED

In the end, Steve easily accepted my father's answer. But many years later, after the scars of our successful surgery had healed, some nights when eating dinner he could never really explain why he had developed a taste for all of the Italian foods I used to love eating at my grandmother's house.

Only the wisest men admit there is so much in this world that we do not know or understand. This story is one of them.

CHAPTER XII

No guts...no glory. This statement was originally intended to aid the intestinal fortitude for a person to do the right thing. The situation I now faced was giving up my guts for another guy's glory.

The operation to harvest my organs had reached the halfway point. There wasn't much left in my lower abdomen except for my intestines and gonads, and I sort of wanted to be buried with my balls still attached. My chest was scheduled to be opened up next and then, as TV detectives always seem to say, we will get to the heart of the matter.

While I laid in bed before I died and the operation had begun, the endless time of televised trivia had taken its toll. Listening to daytime game shows and soap operas had grown worse than boring. I could tell when night arrived as another repeat movie was being shown and then the late night news and talk shows announced another day had passed by.

The only time that my intellect was now perked up was when the nightly and morning news programs expounded on my medical situation. They told of how perseverance and courage still counted for something more than money for my family. Even though my prognosis was still non-productive and terminal, my pathology had begun producing a propensity for extrasensory perceptions. My psyche was gaining daily a preponderance for paranormal remote viewing of me and my room. With my sight and voice and muscles shut down, my mind opened up other doorways of perception. Even though I knew I was being kept alive only by extreme life saving support machinery and understood I would never again talk, react, or move, my mental capacities were increasing in an astral direction that after my final death would help me find my future fate.

So I subconsciously began learning how to adjust and relate to my outer shell's social and physical environment. During this time the recipients and family members and friends continued to flood into my room to pay their last respects or gain some insight about my willfully given gifts.

When the young man named Tom, who was to receive my small intestines was wheeled into my room he looked half dead. His skin was ashen and he had no strength. Tom was bound to his wheelchair with chest straps so he wouldn't fall out and had several I.V. bottles hanging high behind him, which through tubes and connectors were keeping him alive. He had already lived beyond his life expectancy after his initial emergency surgery had given him but a ten percent survival rate of success. He was the same age as me, and it seemed a shame for him to die before he could even vote. In the last attempt to save his life, he was to undergo the extreme experimental surgery where my intestines would be transplanted into him. Last year this surgery was conducted 79 times, but there was no reliable survival data yet available, except he would soon die if he didn't undergo the transplantation.

While I was in school I had been taught that transplant surgery had been conducted since 1823 when a German surgeon performed plastic surgery on a woman's nose by grafting skin from her thigh. The surgical techniques were next greatly improved during the early 20th Century by French researchers. But it wasn't until the 1950's when immunologists discovered the criteria of histocompatibility for tissue matching, that along with the development of immunosuppressive drugs, made transplants more viable. Cyclosporine and tacrolimus had been discovered to have remarkable immunosuppressive properties and revolutionized the transplant market in 1983. So now almost every few years since 1967 when Doctor Barnard conducted the world's first successful heart transplant, the advances of medical science continue to improve. The great strides to implant organs are what Tom was depending upon. He knew in his terminal case that any hope was better than no hope.

He was dying because his viscera were overtaken by a virulent virus. In his poisonous pathogenic state he did not have long to survive. His colon was cancerous and his abdominal organs were no longer functioning due to thousands of polyps. These cylindrical bodyworks were arising inward from his intestines' epithelial lining and far too numerous to be individually removed. The polyps had caused massive blockages of his intestines, which resulted in a swelling of the cecum. This blind sac is located where the small intestine joins the large and has a finger-sized projection called the appendix. He suffered an acute appendicitis attack which quickly became critical and the organ became massively infected and rapidly filled with deadly fluids. Overnight his appendix swelled like a balloon, and when it could stretch no more it burst and caused a serious generalized infection of Tom's abdominal lining called peritonitis.

Tom knew that the small intestine is a long coiled tube connected to the large intestine and is about one half its length, but double in its diameter. At its beginning the intestines are joined to the stomach by the duodenum, and at its other end it delivers undigested wastes and intestinal bacteria to the rectum which connects to the anus. The inner walls of the intestine are circularly ribbed and lined with extremely small finger-like projections called villi. The individual cells on this hair-thin villi structure also have minute projections to increase the surface and absorption of the nutrients and water in the digestive system. If the intestines were smooth walled, they would have to be approximately seven football fields in length to have a comparable surface area.

About ten liters of water each day pass through your intestines. Two of them enter the digestive tract as a result of eating and drinking, and the remaining eight liters carry the various substances secreted by the digestive glands. About 99% of this water is reabsorbed in your intestines. When it isn't reabsorbed, then ion loss, dehydration and diarrhea result.

Tom's intestines were not working at all due to the blockages caused by the cancer and infections. His belly had drastically swollen and only the surgically installed drainage tubes stopped his skin from splitting in two due to the internal pressure of the infected fluids. The doctors were pumping into him massive amounts of vitamins and medicines to help combat the infections, but he still was slipping away from life a little more each day.

It turned out I died just in time to save Tom. He had been operated on the day before me to remove and clean out all of his infected intestines. It was an emergency operation without which he would have died. The doctors then temporarily put a drainage tube into his stomach and tied off his rectum and closed him up with temporary sutures until my intestines were available for transplantation. The next day after I died the doctors disconnected my bowels and taped and superglued them together to retain their shape and size and then removed them as one large package to be implanted within Tom. Without binding the yards of intestines together, they would have uncoiled and been impossible to reassemble within Tom's torso.

This experimental operation was the first time that the small and large intestines were ever transplanted together into a new recipient and made medical history.

To some people this story will seem too incredible to be true. To others that suffer from colon cancer, they only pray that it is true. During the past 50 years transplantation techniques have astronomically improved, and today surgeons do what was undreamed of yesterday.

We all know that life is but an illusion, and death will always be our ultimate reality. But while we are within the land of the living, the lessons we learn prepare us for our path towards paradise.

Only time will tell if Tom will survive, but our story proves that anything can happen when you dare to believe that the life you live can lead on to better ways.

CHAPTER XIII

Having now removed all of my usable organs from my abdominal cavity while the heart and lung machine maintained my dead body's blood pressure and breathing, the transplant teams again changed places. The last eight hours had gone by quickly, and my pulse and respiration had remained regular during the previous surgery's harvesting procedures.

With surgical saws, clamps and spreaders, the next transplant team split apart my breastbone and cut the pericardial members open to expose my heart and lungs. Concurrently, the recipient's chest was also opened and tubes were placed to connect this patient to a heart-lung machine that would keep him alive until my heart is implanted within him. When the team removes his heart, they will leave the upper chamber of his heart in place so they can stitch the new heart onto it. Heart transplants are the third most common implant operation in the U.S.

But again it seems I am getting ahead of the story. I am not trying to rush through this, but after watching my body being dissected during the last eight hours and seeing my parts being implanted into others, it's hard to believe that this surgery is only half done.

The name of the guy who was receiving my heart was Hank, and he was in the fall season of his life. He jokingly said that he had so many bypasses completed that they ought to name a highway after him. Hank didn't think he was really funny, but humor was now his only defense against the deadly situation he faced.

He knew that heart transplants are the most dramatic and perhaps most difficult of all organ transplants. Because once you no longer have a functioning heart, life goes downhill in a hurry. A patient cannot survive on their own without their heart beating for more than a few minutes.

Although price is no object when you are about to die, Hank was well aware of the cost of heart surgery. He had already been billed over $100,000 for previous surgeries, and this transplant would cost over $100,000 more. During the last couple of years while he was waiting with the 4,152 people on the organ recipient list to join the 2,345 people who annually receive heart transplants, along with the bypass surgeries to unblock his veins he also was one of the 60,000 Americans to have implanted pig heart valves to replace his heart's worn out valves. Even after the new xenotransplants healed, he also had to have a manmade artificial organ called a left-ventricular assist device implanted beside his heart. This pump and pacemaker helps his heart to keep the blood flowing and him alive until a donor's heart was available. The treatments and fees were not cheap, but he reasoned that he couldn't take his money to the grave with him and his insurance coverage helped out a lot.

Hank's doctors kept on encouraging him throughout all of his surgeries by reminding him that 84% of heart transplants survive the next year, and most patients are able to resume their normal lives about six months after the implant surgery is completed.

Fifty years old was Hank, and he hoped to live for many more years by his lifelong wife's side watching their six children and sixteen grandchildren grow up. Even though he was in the fall season of his life, his offspring were but in the spring of theirs.

My family already knew Hank because he was a local pharmacist who regularly filled my father's patients' prescriptions. Someone once said that the circle of life is divided into six degrees of separation, but the likelihood of one of my father's professional associates receiving an implant from me seemed much more unusual than that. Our rare AB+ blood types and histocompatibility match were only shared by 3% of Americans, and his chest cavity was large enough for my enlarged swimmer's heart to fit in.

I didn't know until I heard the doctors discussing it, but swimming athletes due to their training and over-exertion while underwater for years of their lives, develop heart ventricles that can be 30% to 50% larger than the normal chambers that our blood is pumped through. Our hearts are the hardest working muscles in our body. It is a muscular organ that is about the size of your fist, and it controls our cardiovascular system. Your heart lies directly behind your breastbone and is encased in the pericardium, which is a thick membranous sac that the fluid within has a lubricating and cushioning effect. The heart is divided into the left side and right and each has an upper and lower chamber. Oxygen-depleted blood comes in the right, then passes to your lungs and then is returned to the left side reinvigorated with oxygen. Next it is pumped throughout your body, and after flowing through your circulatory system is returned depleted of oxygen to the right side of your heart and starts its recycling all over again. The left ventricle has the harder job of pumping blood throughout your entire body, so its muscular walls are thicker than those of the right. The capacity of the left ventricle is about two ounces of blood. Since your heart beats about 70 times a minute, in one hour your heart has moved over 500 pounds of blood. The valves inside of your heart are one way only and do not allow a backward flow of blood. This astral engineering design allows your hard working little heart to push your blood through your aorta and into your carotid, mesenteric, renal, and iliac arteries and their arterioles, capillaries, and veins. If all of these blood vessels were connected end to end, they would extend over 50,000 miles.
    Hank's heart started dying because of hypertension. High blood pressure caused by cholesterol accumulating in his arteries and interfering with the flow of his blood had created this cardiovascular disease which is the leading cause of untimely deaths in the western world. His atherosclerosis began in early adulthood, and Hank's smoking, overweight and poor diet contributed greatly in the degenerative progress until in one artery the fatty plaques had caused a blood clot called a thrombus. One day the clot was dislodged from the artery's wall and it moved along being carried with the blood until it reached a previously partially blocked coronary artery which then became totally blocked because of the thrombus. This is how his first heart attack occurred. The thromboembolism caused a

myocardial infarction, and a portion of his heart muscle died due to the lack of oxygen.

Although he took nitroglycerin and other drugs to dilate his blood vessels, thin his blood, and help relieve the pain, the silent killer of hypertension continued to try and kill him the same way it did his dad and grandfather. The hypercholesterolemia was but part of the problem. Even though helpful measures regarding diet and exercise were originally ordered to help offset his genetic predisposition to the development of his family's hypertension, the occurrence of his heart attacks still slowly increased until only mechanical assistance was now keeping him alive.

Now two years after his first attack of angina pectoris, which racked his chest in raging pain and radiated in his left arm, Hank practiced meditation to reduce stress, did yoga-like stretching, quit smoking, lost weight, and under his physical therapist's guidance did cardiovascular exercises and was now considered medically fit to attempt the heart implantation.

When the big day came, Hank was no longer joking around. He knew this was his last resort at living life amongst his family and friends. He and my father had talked some every day, but on the day I was declared dead, no words could describe the mixed emotions that Hank felt. The contradictory situation of his self-preservation by me perishing would forever influence his remaining days.

Under a general anesthesia, the doctors removed Hank's old heart and left in place the upper atriums which were attached to the pulmonary veins, arteries, superior vena cava and aorta. By leaving the basic plumbing that was attached to the pump of his heart in place, it would greatly facilitate the implantation of his new heart. When my recently removed heart, which was stored in an icepack reached his operating table, the aorta of mine was first attached to his, and then the atriums and supporting blood vessels were also quickly reattached. After the blood vessels were again sealed tight and the stitches that joined our two hearts together as one were proven to be leak resistant, then our heartbeat was re-energized with an injection of fluid which made our heart first burp and then start beating in a regular rhythm again. As the familiar lub-dub sound was heard due to the vibration of the heart's valves, a pulse wave passed down the walls of the arterial blood vessels as the aorta expanded and then recoiled following the ventricle systole. The intrinsic beating of our hearts would now forever be as but one.

As Hank's systolic and diastolic blood pressure measurements became normalized, his breastbone was wired back together and his incision was closed using layers of stitches to sew his muscles and skin back together again. If the graft rejection could be controlled, his survival would be increased up to an additional ten years.

Months of physical and drug therapy passed before Hank's heart allowed him to live a new life. During these days my dad visited with him at the end of his hospital rounds. They talked a little about everything and some days about nothing at all. In time, Hank's contradictory continuum of consciousness was slowly soothed by a contrite and consolatory convergence.

After this happened, during one of his conversations with my father Hank revealed his homage to what a hero he thought I was. He told my dad that to save another's life while yours is ending is what Medals of Honor are presented for. Then Hank continued to expound on and explain, that even if the rest of the world did not recognize what a distinguished award I was due, that once I reached paradise my own personal reward would be to truly know that to die a good death is the most esteemed and worthy of endings to life.

It wasn't until now that I learned the Lord's loftiest lesson, that the sharing of my flesh helped lead to the salvation of my soul.

So please learn to live every day as if it will be your last…because one day it will be. Your name and deeds are the only things that continue to live on after you die. Please, please make them both count for the greater good.

CHAPTER XIV

But I still wasn't finished with learning the lessons of the living. My lungs would be the next organ transplanted from me into a lad named Larry.

With each of my implants came a clearer sense of caring and an improved clarity of the universal cyclopedic cusp of curing. As the hours of the operation continued to pass by, I continued to discover that being dead isn't nearly as bad as you might think compared to some of the diseases you could live with.

Larry's lungs had been destroyed by asbestos. This carcinogenic causing agent that had poisoned his place of work ruined his respiratory system due to his long-term inhalation of asbestos fibers that were coated with metallic and mineral dusts. This case just goes to show that most people never understand the dangers in their workplace until they are almost dead.

Even black lung disease or tuberculosis would have been kinder diseases that he stood a chance of correcting, than the pneumoconiosis he suffered due to the characterizations of the chemical agents he inhaled.

Your lungs work together to bring oxygenated air in contact with your blood and carry away carbon dioxide. The breathing passageways and lungs resemble an upside-down tree covered with two cone-shaped, spongy organs resembling balloons in function and form. Your respiratory tract extends from the nose to the lungs, which lie deep within the thoracic cavity behind your rib cage and above your diaphragm where they are protected from drying out. As air moves through your nose, pharynx, trachea and the bronchi, it is then divided towards your two lungs. There it is filtered, warmed and humidified. Once in your lungs the air is warmed to body temperature and saturated with water as it continues its path through your smaller passageways called bronchioles, which subdivide many, many times, and then terminates in an elongated space resembling a bunch of microscopic grapes which enclose a multitude of air pockets called alveoli. Once the air is there, a gas exchange occurs between it and your blood as carbon dioxide leaves and oxygen enters the blood and combines with hemoglobin in the red blood cells. This is why the quality of the environmental air which Larry breathed in pollutants had poisoned his life.

By inhaling particles of asbestos he contracted pulmonary fibrosis in which the fibrous bodies built up in his lungs and impaired his breathing capacity. Because of the constant irritation, the small hair-like cilia that lined his upper respiratory tract dried out and died and no longer functioned as a screening device. After they went through a degenerative change, the cilia lost their air cleaning ability and chronic bronchitis infected his lungs.

His frequent coughing soon damaged and collapsed the bronchioles which then trapped old air in his alveoli. Without renewed air, these extremely small grape bunched balloons lost their elasticity and soon ruptured. The emphysema he now suffered made Larry breathless because the surface area of his lungs was greatly reduced and not enough oxygen reached his heart and brain.

This long-term chain reaction resulted in his constant coughing and made his heart work faster forcing more blood through his damaged system and made him feel depressed, sluggish, and irritable.

Now because his breathing capacity was so seriously impaired, along with drug therapy, the doctors induced one lung at a time to collapse. This painful pneumothorax procedure was intended to allow one lung enough time to heal while the other did double duty at respiration.

But Larry's condition worsened as the cells lining his bronchi continued to thicken and callus. It now was impossible for his body to prevent dust and dirt from settling in his lungs and soon atypical nuclei appeared in the callused lining. These cancerous disordered cells finally broke lose and penetrated other tissues. The metastasis continued to migrate until it formed a tumor which blocked a bronchus and totally cut off the supply of air to one lung.

His lung now collapsed on its own weight and the secretions trapped within became infected and localized areas of pus resulted. Next pneumonia caused by the bacterium infected his lung and the lobules became totally non-functional as they filled up with fluid.

The surgeons next elected to remove that lung completely before any secondary growths had time to form. After this pneumonectomy operation, Larry was left with only half of his original 300 million alveoli and no defense mechanisms to limit future microbe invasions of his body.

Massive drug therapy to deter other tumors now was even further enhanced, and the targeted therapies to help hold the disease in place, along with standard chemotherapy, resulted in the side effect symptoms of shortness of breath, exhaustion, coughs, poor appetite, nausea, and some increased risk of other infections and cancers because his immune system was put out of order and he no longer had a source of white blood cells to protect against future infections. He even underwent the surgical experimental implantation of the BioLung. This plastic pencil length artificial organ consisted of two accordion tubes packed with micropores and attached to his heart and an outside plastic lung. The artificial lung was only meant as a temporary bridge until a human donation was available and the device carried the risk of infections.

But when you are dying a little every day and have already lost one lung, you aren't too worried about getting any germs or catching a cold next month or even another form of cancer. When each breath you take may be your last, you live life but a heartbeat at a time.

It is projected that between 1990 and 2020 almost two million deaths could be caused by unwarranted asbestos exposure in the workplace. Lung transplants are hampered by the extreme difficulty in preserving the lungs from a recently deceased person that are still usable until a matching recipient is found. Last year approximately 900 lungs were transplanted in the United States with a 75% one year survival rate. There are over 4,000 people on the waiting list and millions more in the shadow of death not knowing when asbestos or another abnormality will cause a deadly disease or disorder to claim their life.

When Larry came to the hospital he couldn't walk or talk. He was moved in a wheelchair and could only breathe using a mask supplying oxygen enriched air. Even with these and other devices he could barely stay awake. He needed a double lung transplant or he would die. With a shaky hand he wrote notes to my family, which they read aloud while his wife cried tears of hurt and hope. With every breath Larry took, he could only pray it wasn't his last.

His wife told us of their long evaluation procedure to determine if he was the most appropriate candidate for treatment. His age and general health were two of the most important considerations. Since at the age of thirty he had one foot in the coffin and his other not far behind, and his other organs had not yet been infected, the medical specialists determined his strength was sufficient to survive the surgery. His AB+ blood type as well as his body size also matched mine, and his rare blood type proved most beneficial because as I may have said before only 3% of the U.S. male population shared in this matching.

Most lung transplants are single-lungs, but because Larry already had one of his lungs removed due to his infectious lung disease and had undergone massive medication, the pulmonary rehabilitation team, which consisted of doctors who specialize in cardiology, infectious disease, transplant surgery, anesthesiology, psychiatry, nutrition and social and physical rehabilitation, made a comprehensive assessment and decided it would be best for Larry to undergo a double transplant. This care didn't come cheap. In addition to the $250,000 of previous medical treatments, his surgery would exceed another $250,000. He would also remain in the hospital for the next three to six months until he was fully recovered at the cost of $1,500 per day for nursing care and medications. And then for the remainder of his life he would undergo follow-up blood tests and x-rays and take anti-rejection medications. All in all, the cost to recover his life due to the asbestos poisoning would exceed $2 million, which was to be paid by his union's insurance coverage.

When he was first admitted to the hospital, Larry was assigned a primary nurse, who in addition to the operating room, intensive care unit, thoracic care unit and the rehabilitation staff, would coordinate his care plan in the hospital and home.

The day I died Larry was immediately transferred to the operating room where an anesthesiologist prepared him for surgery. He was connected to a cardiopulmonary bypass machine which would assist his heart and breathing during the next ten hours of surgery.

After the surgeons removed my lungs and declared them fit for transplantation, an incision was cut side to side across the lower part of Larry's chest. His old lung was removed through this opening after it was disconnected from his pulmonary artery and veins and the main stem bronchus. His diaphragm was next lowered and my pair of lungs, which are naturally curved on the back surface to have room for the heart, esophagus, trachea, and blood vessels, were reconnected to Larry's blood and air supply ways and then fitted into his collarbone and ribs and filled up his chest cavity. The incisions were next closed and a dressing applied to the opening that will take several uncomfortable weeks to heal.

After the surgery was completed, Larry immediately was given several immuno-suppressive medications to help prevent rejection and special precautions were taken to prevent infections. For weeks anyone entering his room would be required to wear a gown, gloves, and mask to insure communicable complications did not occur. Soon after his surgery he resumed physical therapy activities and eating a good nutritional diet. His days were regulated by therapy, testing, and rest and recuperation periods.

Even with all of these precautions and support mechanisms, his three-year survival statistics were only a 50/50 chance of still being alive. Because having a deadly disease which causes a lung transplant is bound to be emotionally difficult for both the patient and family members, there are extensive emotional support systems in place which provide nursing staff, social workers, psychiatric help and patient transplant support groups that hold regular meetings to discuss questions or problems that may arise. But Larry knew he was lucky to be alive instead of joining the 80% of lung failure patients who die while 13 million more people who suffer some form of chronic lung disease await their end-stage failure.

Months later during one of these support meetings Larry was

discussing with another transplant patient about how he knew his life could be short, but what a wonderful feeling it was to be able to take a single breath and not fall over wheezing in agony; that to be able to walk on his own two legs instead of being wheeled about was a sensation he didn't just a few months ago ever believe he would have again experienced; of how his life had changed in so many positive ways; and how he prayed each day that his donor could somehow experience his energetic exhalations and hear of him receiving a new lease on life.

It is time to let you know that I believe while telling this story I may be repeating myself. I don't mean to do so. It is as if the lights are on in my head, but the voltage is low and I am slowly growing dull in this state of existence. So please pardon me as I try to reach out and touch you with my story. It does mean much more to me than our skin's sense of touch transmitting pressure, pleasure, or pain.

I so wanted to touch Larry and let him know that not only could I feel his prayers, but I also experienced his improvements. What was mine is now his, and what was his is now mine. Over the forthcoming years we came to understand that together, with each breath we took for the remainder of our conjoined days, we both would know that there are but two great loves in life…what you do with it and who you do it with.

CHAPTER XV

The transplant team had again been replaced with a fresh group of surgeons that would next be removing my eyes. It was then after the transplantation of my corneas was completed that I realized I grew up never really seeing myself as I really was.

Edward was scheduled to receive my implants which during surgery would transplant my clear corneas to replace his. The most frequent causes of loss of vision are, in order, retinal disorders, glaucoma and cataracts, and only 4% of blindness results from injuries. Edward's disability was in the minority.

While he was working on polishing a piece of a brass casting he had created during an art studio class in college, the buffing machine he was using had a wire wheel disintegrate and accidentally showered his face with thousands of small wires. These shards were razor sharp, and due to his failure to wear safety goggles, the wires not only imbedded in his facial skin, but hundreds of microscopic pieces of metal also pierced both of his eyes.

The corneas of his eyes, which are the clear front windshield and the strongest focusing lens, were totally destroyed in the accident and the scleral tissue that forms the white of his eyes became infected. Also his nose, lips and skin were pierced more times than a porcupine. Although there was no cause to laugh at his dumbness and distress, as the disorder permanently blinded him. The irony was that in pursuit of his art for others to see, he lost both of his eyes.

Normal vision depends on your cornea staying clear, smooth, and thin. The pieces of metal wires had caused cloudy spots on his lens and eventually a secondary infection pervaded the whole lens. This turned his clear lens a milky shade of yellow-white. His cornea next lost its clarity because it was severely swollen and scarred, the incoming light became scattered and blocked his vision.

After microsurgery, which used a magnet to help withdraw the shards, many medications were used to try to limit the amount of visual loss, but the damage was too severe and the medicine could not clear his vision.

Six months ago Edward's surgical team decided that a corneal transplant should be considered to correct his vision. They informed him and his family that all surgery has some inherent risks. No transplant can ever be expected to give as good a result as the original organ. But corneal transplants do help the 33,000 people every year that elect to undergo this reconstructive eye surgery technique, with a success rate greater than 90 percent.

The eye doctors continued to explain to his family that the surgery, which was developed in the 1950's, was one of the earliest tissue transplantations. The most common form of corneal transplants is penetrating keratoplasty, during which the central segment of a full thickness cornea is replaced by donor tissue. The success rate has improved dramatically during the past 50 years due to improved tissue culture selection, storage techniques, and vastly increased skills of operating room personnel using new instrumentation and operating microscopes that utilize lasers to assure precise cutting of the corneas of the donor and recipient. These refined techniques minimize tissue inflammation and provide rapid recovery due to reduced postoperative complications.

When Edward was led into my room, my mother gasped in shock because he was the same age and general appearance as me. She couldn't stop staring as my dad and the hospital's transplant team explained the total surgical procedure of what was to happen to me the day I died.

My mother was again openly crying aloud as they explained to Edward that his surgery would occur towards the end of the procedure, because the tissue culture system would permit storage of my corneas for several days if need be. But for the best outcome, the transplant would be completed as soon as possible after the other organs that were more time lapse susceptible had been harvested.

When the transplant team was through with their explanation of the events, they asked Edward if he had any questions. I could hear a strange quirk in his voice as he said he did. Edward went on to explain that his mother had read to him most all of the available information about the eyes and their structure and how they sensed light. But what he wanted to first ask was how the focusing function of the eye lens re-righted the inverted images and the backwards words formed on the rear wall of the retina.

By now I had grown used to the fact that everyone who became ill seemed to research their disease or distortion to the dimension of a doctorial term paper. But as I listened to the conversation, his technical question didn't sound as silly as when I first heard it.

My dad asked Edward to explain what he knew about the focusing of the eye. With a scholar's sense of showmanship, he started with the basics, explaining that light rays enter the eye and are bent when they pass through the cornea and then refracted by the lens and finally brought into focus on the retina. To focus on distant or near objects, the ciliary muscle remains relaxed or contracted to allow the lens to remain rounded or flattened when the ligaments become taut. The light rays that emit from each point of the object being viewed are bent by the cornea and lens in such a way that they cross at a single midway point and continue onto the rear wall of the retina, but now being projected inverted.

Edward took a breath and continued on saying that it was the same image that took place in a telescope or at the rear wall of a camera. He knew the refraction of the projected image appearing on the inner retina wall was rotated 180° from the actual and appeared as an inverted image and the field of vision was reversed in a mirror image. So now in your eye everything was reversed and upside down and would appear as crazy as holding this book upside down in front of a mirror and trying to read the pages from the reflection.

As Edward paused it was obvious that the medical team was initially expecting more of a question about color blindness, astigmatism, eye color or corneal transplant rejections, but when there was but a silent stillness in the air after his summary of his knowledge about the field of focus, he hesitantly rephrased his question. He simply stated that he wanted to know how people could read things that are projected as bassackwards and upside down.

After recovering their professional demeanor, the ophthalmologist was the first to answer and said in medical school during an experiment he and other students attended during a scientists' study, that they actually wore glasses which reversed and inverted their vision. In the beginning they all had problems adjusting to the placement of objects, but they soon became regulated to life in an upside down and backwards world. He continued on stating many people have taught themselves how to read upside down across a desk from someone who had a confidential file in front of them, and some people can even write in a reversed mirror image with just a little practice. He closed by saying that experiments such as these suggest that although images are perceived reversed and inverted, that your brain has learned to see them right side up and non-reversed.

Edward retorted in a lengthy statement. "But no one knows this for sure. Just as some people's sense of seeing paranormal perceptions or an expanded electromagnetic spectrum encompassing the ultraviolet rays gives them extraordinary viewing power, and some people can give forth an evil eye of a look, or others that are sensitive to people's Chaka colors can measure modes of behavior or even some who can see into the future...the functioning of the eye still remains a mystery. From the ancient masons whose third eye of torah that could envision the past, present and future as one, to the modern medical marvels of today, we continue to push the boundaries of what we perceive from science fiction into fact." He closed by saying that he believed that these perceptions can be enhanced. "The same way you learn in the spectrum of colors that white is the absence of color and black is the absorption of all, the existence of clear is a lesson that is perceived not by normal color differentiation, but rather by touch. Until as a child you learn to reach out to determine if a clear pane of glass is in front of you, then you just keep on bumping into it until you or it breaks."

The room grew quiet after Edward's statement, but if I could have, I would have yelled out an amen. I knew firsthand that the limits we perceive aren't all there is to see. Many times it seems that life doesn't hold as much meaning as we think it should. Then you die and see events with a new sense of sight and discover things that before were invisible to human eyes.

As the day of my surgery continued on, Edward's dream to see again came true. The corneas of my eyes were removed and since I was already pre-screened for AIDS, syphilis, and hepatitis, the doctors knew that they were fit for transplantation. Next my corneas were placed in a special storage liquid until it was time for Edward's surgery.

His surgery was done under a local anesthetic with his eyes numbed with a Novocain-like medicine, but he would remain awake. Using a special round cutting tool called a trephine, his diseased corneas were removed one at a time. After my corneas were cut to a matching size, they were placed in his eyes and secured in place with very small, fine stitches. The corneas were transplanted in such a manner that no blood vessels came in contact with them, and therefore the body could not send immune cells through the blood vessels to attack the new corneas. His surgery would take six to nine months to heal, and until then the stitches would not be removed and medicated eye drops would be used against allograft reaction and to make sure the transplants heal properly.

At the end of a year, Edward returned to college to eat, drink, breathe, smell and see the all American dream come true. But for the rest of his days on earth he could never look in a mirror and see life only through his own point of view. For he did discover that when dreams and desires inspire the daring to do, that the impossible becomes the improbable and then becomes the provable.

With his new sense of sight he knew that God's will is not the collection of riches or the possession of power. He decided to get real with his religion, for he could now see with absolute clarity that all the paths we choose will eventually and always lead to the grave. So why not choose a righteous one?

CHAPTER XVI

Make no bones about it, by the time the ninth surgical team was assembled by my bedside I knew that everyone was becoming a winner. There would be no losers in this game of give and take, except your ears being exposed to my bone-dry humor.

The next person to get a second chance at life was Bob. Although it was really his third chance. At 50 years old he was originally diagnosed with colon cancer, but the disease was detected very early on during an annual medical exam. The bone he had to pick on was that while the cancer had been brought under remission with surgery, drug therapy, and intensive chemotherapy, the radiation treatments had destroyed his bone marrow along with the cancerous cells. Bob hadn't been born bad to the bone, and because of my bones he wouldn't be buried before his time in a bone yard either.

Bob did not have a cantankerous bone in his body, but his bone of contention was without a transplant to replace the production of his blood stem cells which had been killed off, he would remain in a life-threatening situation. The only hope for a cure would be a bone marrow transplant to replace his diseased cells with healthy, new cells.

I knew from my college studies that the bone of truth was that bone marrow is the living tissue found in the center of bone spaces filled with spongy looking bars and plates that are separated by irregular spaces. Although lighter than compact bones, the solid portions of spongy bones follow lines of stress and are designed to add strength. The medullary cavity inside of long bones contains yellow bone marrow, and the spongy bones located beneath the cartilage at the larger ends of long bones and flat bones, such as the skull, ribs, breastbone, scapula, and the pelvic coxal bones, are filled with red bone marrow. Yellow bone marrow is a fat storage tissue and red bone marrow produces stem cells. Very special cells called stem cells are developed in the red bone marrow and are the source for red and white blood cells, which are the primary forces of the immune system.

Every blood cell in the bone marrow starts its life as a stem cell which then divides and forms the different cells that compose your blood and immune system. Your white cells fight against infections and the red cells carry oxygen and clotting agents. The bare-bone explanation is that without bone marrow your immune system is severely impaired and you could die from a cold or even any common infection.

Blood stem cells can be harvested from three different sources, of which each has its benefits and risks. Bone marrow is a very rich source of blood stem cells and has a history of over 13,000 documented donor transplants, and more scientific data has been collected than other treatments due to its extensive use. Your bloodstream is also another source of stem cells, but to have enough cells regularly available, a special growth factor drug called filgrastim must be given to the patient before the donor undergoes a process called apheresis. During these sessions the stem cells are separated from the donor's enriched blood without the need for an anesthesia, and the remaining blood is returned back to their bloodstream. The first successful transplant using peripheral blood stem cells occurred during 1986. But some studies show that this type of transplant engraft can result in a chronic phenomenon known as graft-versus-host disease. This is when the transplanted stem cells start to make white blood cells, and the blood production from these donated stem cells attacks the patient's body. The third source is from a full-term baby's umbilical cord, which is collected at birth, tissue-typed, processed and then stored frozen until needed. This accepted medical practice was first done in 1988, and negative detriments include the small fixed amount of stem cells available are sometimes not enough for a patient. Also there is a chance that a genetic disease might be transmitted through the umbilical cord that other marrow and blood donors' genetic disorders can be pre-screened for. On the positive side, there is no donor risk or pain to mother or child, and post-transplant risks are less, which allows for less than perfect match ups between donor and the recipient.

We knew in our bones for any transplant to be successful the cells of each must match as closely as possible. Bone marrow exchanges require a closer matching of donor and recipient than any other type of transplant. About one out of three patients who require a bone marrow transplant have a close family member who as an allogeneic live donor is suitably matched.

But Bob's options were bone dry since his only brother had already passed away, as well as his mother and father. The reason he joined the U.S. list of 1,500 people waiting to undergo an unrelated allogeneic bone marrow transplant whose chances of success are less than 50/50, is that he wanted to watch his children grow up for as long as he could. The doctors had caught his cancer early and forced it into remission. Now the only way he could continue to live after having his bone marrow destroyed, was replacing it with new marrow that didn't produce the faulty blood cells.

You couldn't tickle Bob's funny bone as the donor match for him became more difficult. His family even considered that since they couldn't control the length of the waiting list, perhaps it would be a good time to control what they could. They then began to educate themselves about an alternative experimental treatment for infusion of embryonic stem cells. These cells are found in the very early stages of human embryos and appear capable of developing into almost any type of cell in the human body. Although ethical issues and questions haunt this field of study, the intensive donor solicitations of the past decade have not made much of a dent in the backlog of usable organs and tissue for transplantation. The implantation or creation of organs and tissues from aborted fetuses has faced huge opposition. Although some researchers have collected these inner cells and cultured them in the laboratory and developed specialized cells that show great promise for improving the survival rates for awaiting transplant patients.

As luck had it, my death and excellent histocompatibility with Bob's ended his immediate endangerment, and his ethics didn't have to bear scrutiny. But the bone of truth is that there is still a whole lot of science and medical hocus pocus that will have to come into play to produce the one liter of usable bone marrow for a stem cell transplant.

The red bone marrow was removed from my bones during surgery using needles and syringes to suck out the marrow from the inner spongy cavities. The next procedure that could produce the best outcome was somewhat experimental. Because of our unrelated bone marrow transfer, our partially matched human lymphocyte-associated complex proteins could be improved by removing the T lymphocytes from my stem cells.

There would never be a bone of contention between us because to reduce the chances of rejection, the cytotoxic T-cells, which are sometimes called "killer T-cells" that attack or trigger antibodies into cleansing infectious organisms or their toxins, would first be removed from my immune system's response. After the researchers withdrew the T-cells' mediated immunity to search out and destroy antigen-bearing cells, the scientists next would activate the cells by culturing them in the presence of the recipient's interleukins. These are messenger molecules produced by either your lymphocytes or monocytes and then these reacclimated customized killer cells are reinjected into the patient. Now the production of blood by the new recipient stem cells is recognized as the original. The killer cells are fooled and can't recognize the new cells as foreigners and won't attack the new host's body, thus autoimmune illnesses are avoided and the T-cells won't try to kill off the new body's tissues.

Although we both started out as individuals as unique as a fingerprint, during Bob's and my forthcoming years together our major complex proteins and genes were continuously intra-traded. Years later after our conjoining grew continuously more complex and the D.N.A. of mine was thoroughly intermixed with his, I often wondered if some of his stray thoughts or automatic responses weren't some of the memories of everything I was or about to be.

But you have to forgive my boneheaded attempt to be comical or funny in a death defying situation. My punning is not particularly funny. Nor does my word play on a bone-dry life and death situation appear with an anatomic trace of humor...unless your funny bone feels humerus.

CHAPTER XVII

I hadn't yet grown thin skinned during my operation. Matter of fact, my soul felt strong and my spirit was still stretching by being extended into the seekers of my donated organs.

I forget if I may have said before, but it is a well documented fact that as you lose some of your body's sensory sensations, the remaining senses you have become more accurate and acute. A blind man hears very well. A deaf and mute individual's vision becomes eagle like. A quadriplegic's mind expands beyond its original limits. Now, imagine losing all of your earthly senses and what remains to be expanded may be beyond your imagination.

My sense of time had now become as fluid as a pool of water. I could drift about in time or choose to swim forward or backwards at any speed I wished. But this swimming pool had no end or beginning and I never grew tired while swimming. I began to realize that my celestial chariot was being presented to me in the most common medium that I was accustomed to. And since I had spent half of my life in swimming pools, this would become my mode of traveling in time.

Now while within my pool of perception I could travel in seven different directions. I could move aligned in the compassed measured angles of north, south, east and west, or orientate myself up and down, or even at my choosing I could move myself in the seventh most divine direction...which is within. From this celestial center position I was capable of receiving signals from the ten spirits who shared in my flesh. With a smile on my soul's face, I knew we all were made of stars.

I could join up with the people who were implanted with my parts in the present or preview the future, but not the past. That direction was reserved for my memories of the time before we were conjoined. I could regress into my own past and see again my father and grandfather proudly standing together at my high school graduation; my mother and grandmother slaving over huge Sunday dinners and my sisters doing the dishes; and even see my dog who grew up with me and was protective against anyone who wasn't in our family.

Sometimes I even caught obscure hints from members of my club of ten that realized a sense of me, similar to a deja vu or dualistic thought, was within what they were doing or thinking. But I often wondered if anyone else other than them had an inkling that my spirit was still alive and well with them.

Sammy helped provide me that answer, but there I go again getting ahead of myself. You all don't know yet that Sammy is the hometown boy who received my skin.

Just three weeks ago this local ten-year-old boy was playing with his brothers in the family's garage during one bad day when the rainy weather was too harsh to be outside. He accidentally ran his bicycle into a storage shelf that toppled over on top of him. Some containers then broke open and spilled flammable fluids that were doused on him. The liquids were next ignited by the pilot light of the hot water heater which flashed the fluids afire. This accident caused Sammy, who was trapped beneath the metal shelving, to lose over fifty percent of his skin. He was lucky though that the fire was on his lower body, and his lungs had escaped the flames. Otherwise, he could have been charred to death from the inside out.

Each year over 50,000 people are hospitalized for burn treatment. Many of them are children who suffer or die from burn related accidents. Fires cause over 5,500 deaths each year and are one of the greatest hazards of growing up during childhood. Since the 1960's the medical attention for improving the expertise in the burn care field has greatly improved, and the expanded treatment and medical care has spawned research centers for severely burned children.

Since these first specialized burn care units opened, the survival rate for children with burns over fifty percent of their bodies has doubled.

So advanced are the medical burn treatments that many patients who would have in the past certainly died, now survive due to today's improved surgical skills and procedures, expanded medical technology, and the total coordinated efforts of many doctors, nurses and hospital staff members.

It was this multi-hospital's coordinated effort to save Sammy's life that brought this ten-year-old boy into this operating room. Sammy's specialists, surgeons, and his mother and father decided to assist in my family's effort to publicly increase the awareness of the need for national organ and tissue donations.

It was quickly decided that the story of our skin graft would be the tenth in the newspaper's series intended to increase the public's awareness of the ultimate skin game. The reporters' initial written words explained that skin grafting is a surgical procedure of which the first reliable report of was in 1823, when a German surgeon named Carl Bunger grafted skin from a woman's thigh to her nose as reconstructive plastic surgery. This type of skin transplant is called an autograft and avoids problems with rejection.

The reporters went on to explain the other techniques of skin grafting include donated skin called an allograft, animal skin from pigs called xenografts, and several artificial skin products consisting of a synthetic epidermis and a collagen-based dermis. All temporary skin barriers are eventually replaced with a tissue engineered skin grown in the laboratory by culturing the patient's own skin epithelial cells on an artificial surface or the transplantation of the victim's own healthy skin tissues.

Allografts and xenografts provide a temporary skin covering which is extremely important for the recovery of burn patients. Once scars start to form in the affected area, regrowth cannot happen. Skin grafts encourage the serum in the injured skin to ooze out and the healthy cells regenerate the damaged skin. Of the three alternatives, donated skin provides superior protection against infections until the new skin grows back in place.

Large burn wounds that are left on their own will badly scar and actually prevent the movement of limbs. Without the surgical graft of my skin, Sammy would never walk again or could even lose his legs to infection and result in a possible amputation. With the skin graft there would be significant improvement in the burn site healing and would help prevent any serious complications in his recovery.

The article went on to say that the skin is the largest organ of the human body and is sometimes called the integumentary system. Your skin consists of two layers called the epidermis and the dermis. The upper epidermis is a very thin layer of dead cells which provides a tough outer coating derived from the rapid continuous division of cells called keratinocytes. The lower dermis is about ten times as thick as the upper and contains hair follicles, sebaceous glands, sweat glands, blood vessels, receptors, nerve fibers, and the connective tissue called the protein collagen, which provides flexibility and structural support.

To replace Sammy's lost skin, two grafting techniques would be used. Where the wound wasn't too deep, a split-thickness graft would use mainly the upper epidermis and a little of the dermis by using a surgical tool called a dermatome. This technique would allow rapid healing of the burn site cells by his blood vessels nourishing the grafted tissue. In the areas where the damage was much more severe, a full-thickness graft would be used to provide better contour and less contraction at the grafted site. Even after our allografts would be completed, Sammy would still have to undergo a series of other operations using bio-engineered tissues or split-thickness autografts to replace the temporary barrier of the second skin.

After Sammy's skin grafts were in place he would remain in bed for the next weeks with his legs elevated. Then for months he would have to take medication to prevent drying and cracking and to control infectious diseases. He would also undergo hormonal treatments because burned male patients no longer produce testosterone.

Although, as a surprise to everyone, it appeared he did inherit a gene of mine that no one would have ever expected. You would have to be thick skinned to not understand that when drive and determination extend beyond death, next begins a duty of declaring that what is right…is only right. It is then that dreams, desires and the daring to do, evolve into a dogma of devotion.

So the philosophy of the *"we in thee"* allowed me the prospicience prophesy of seeing into the future of Sammy and me. It was while I was within my dues ex machina that I discovered my spirit was still being seen, or at least sensed, by others.

After our operation was over I found myself back again in my pool of perception. I swam forward in time to when a couple of seasons had passed and Sammy's skin grafts were considered a success. I couldn't help but want to see what was happening with him and me. But I was really surprised when I saw his mother and father and him together at my folks' home.

Sammy's parents believed it was a medical miracle that he could again walk and wanted to share their joy with their benefactors. My folks and family had never met Sammy because when he was initially admitted after his accident he was kept in absolute isolation to protect against all forms of infections. Until Sammy had gotten under my skin and his healing had properly commenced, he was confined in quarantine. Now months had passed and due to the rigid physical therapy program and drug treatments, he could again walk with crutches. The first thing he said that he wanted to do was go out and thank my family for giving him a second chance at life.

We lived in the same town so the travel time was short, but the distance between the mindsets of the parents was great. Sammy's parents were glad he was still alive and could walk, and mine were still grieving over my death. My grandparents and sisters still walked about as if at a funeral wake. Even my old dog, Benji, who grew up with me, seemed to have grown bitter and now had taken to barking and biting at all of the strangers who came to our home.

While I was growing up my dog was always protective of me and slept in my room, even when I went away to college. My family even snuck him into the hospital while I was in my coma, hoping his presence would help revive me. But now it was as if my dog sensed my family's despair over my death and intended to keep away any other grief that might show up at their front door.

Sammy's parents had called ahead to pay their regrets and to ask my folks to allow them and their son an opportunity to visit, and now the time and day they agreed upon had arrived.

My dad had already put Benji in the fenced backyard because the dog had tried to attack a mailman a few days before. It was only by the skin of his teeth that Benji hadn't bit the stranger. It was apparent to my folks that they were soon going to have to do something about the dog's behavior, as his defensiveness was escalating into an offensive situation.

When Sammy's parents arrived it took a little while for them to get out of their car because of maneuvering Sammy and his crutches in place. The dog was attentively watching them through the fence slats. With spit flying off from his fangs he had begun barking as soon as their car had come to a stop.

As I watched, the scene soon became chaotic as my mother and father came out of the front door to welcome Sammy's family to their home. The image I next saw would amaze me for the rest of my time.

Benji suddenly stopped barking and put his nose high in the air to better inhale the scent he was seeking. In his eyes was a sense of wild excitement and with but a single jump he cleared the back fence and began running towards the wind that brought a distinctively familiar odor his direction. His loud barking took a new sound of recognition as he bounded towards Sammy.

I couldn't turn my eyes away as my father also took off in a run trying to intercept the dog that appeared to be attacking the family. My father's anxious yells of warning coupled with the dog's insistent barking startled Sammy's frightened family who now were on the sidewalk halfway to the front stoop of our home. As Sammy's mother turned towards the dog, the action appeared to me as if underwater in slow motion. It was apparent that my dog would reach the scared boy before anyone could intervene in the incident. My dog was driven by a quest to hunt down and capture the familiar odor that was recognized by his cunning sense of smell.

I reached out my will to help calm Sammy just as the dog jumped up upon his chest. As my thoughts reached his the boy's terrified expression then changed to compassion. Next his crutches flew aside and Sammy fell on his bottom in the soft grass with the dog standing over him. Benji stopped and stood as still as a stone. Then his tail stood straight up and his nose went to working double time in an effort to determine why my characteristic smell was now being emitted by Sammy. I now understood that somehow my skin had transferred my scent to Sammy. Although dogs see in black and white, they super sensitively smell in a color beyond human perception.

With bated breath Sammy's parents and mine next watch Benji's snarls turn into a smile. His hunt for me was now over. Although he didn't understand why this small boy did not look like me, he knew for sure that the scent he secreted was mine. Like a personal perfume my dog perceived my smell coming from Sammy. And as Benji's tail started wagging excitedly from side to side, he next laid down by Sammy. The look on my old dog's face then turned into a grin of finding a long lost friend.

We all know there is nothing more honest than a smile on a dog's face. Dogs have no reason to deceive us or lie. The scent Benji smelled was more than an indication or hint of my survival. To him, it was positive proof that again I came back home to his side.

It was now that I understood that all of us need to be remembered for what we did, and not what we didn't do. Don't wake up dead one day and say, "I wish I would have done that." Become as one with the wisdom of the *"we in thee"*. Let your soul soar and your spirit grow by donating your shell of skin to someone who will die without a second chance to live out their life's dreams.

CHAPTER XVIII

So it wasn't until after all of the operations were over that I learned the final lesson that the Lord had wanted me to discover about my organ donations. It turned out that the reports of my death had been greatly exaggerated, for now we all know that my spirit lived on within the ten lives touched by mine.

Some skeptics or sociologists may say, "How can this be so?" But all true believers know that faith is a belief beyond facts, fiction or fairy tales.

All of the transplantations were successful and next I was beginning my timeless travels through terrestrial and transcendental theosophies. I would never grow tired of my pursuit of the philosophies of the *"we in thee"*.

In seeking a closure to a story without an end, I first returned to my funeral. It was here I would leave behind the emptied outer shell of skin I had lived within. As the final fantasy of my flesh would end, my spirit flew free and my soul expanded to encompass the ecstasy of a life everlasting.

To prepare my path to paradise and assist my family and friends to accept my accession, the preachers and spokespeople at my funeral made stirring and inspirational speeches. They told of my living achievements, and of at my death, the ultimate gift of giving new lives to ten others who could have died without my donations. It seemed to me that the eulogies were endless and by the closing prayers I wanted to shout out and scream to please listen to me.

I wasn't dead! I had learned to defeat death with my deeds and dogma. No one needs to die in vain, when through your organ donations you can witness a new golden dawn of our world evolving into the next celestial century. When you learn to live to fight, and not have to fight to live, then you will see life for what it really is.

Some people in charge of donor programs were worried that the media exposure grand-standing my gifts of life would increase the use of the news media, magazines, television or the internet to solicit for personal organ donations. That these high profile donors or suave solicitors could try to steer a transplant from the sick or a saint to someone who is popular in print. While it is illegal to sell or pay for an organ in the United States, many people still fear that martyrhood, money or the media exposure caused by launching a marketing campaign could corrupt their system. To these life and death decision makers I can only ask which is worse, to stand by silently and watch hundreds of people die every hour of the day due to the lack of organ donations, or hope that any form of motivation by multi-media exposure may end up saving millions of people's needless suffering or death?

People of this plundered planet are sick and tired of being sick and tired, but not yet ill enough to stop the insanities inspiring the illnesses. Random as rain and as restless as rot or rust, the needless deaths of tens of thousands of people needing organ transplants continues on.

So my prayer from beyond the grave is, please don't wait until you are almost dead before you consider changing your concept of caring. An astral alternative is an ascription to the Almighty which allows you to anew your awareness of avowed answers to amazement, astonishment and awe. Deliver yourself from dying daily a dulled dreary death and instead end your ills by experiencing the enlightenment to which you are truly transcendentally tethered to. Discover a karma of awareness that antedates the cosmic creation and is connected to your consciousness. Once you give the gift of life you are in the grace of God, and guaranteed in your gift of goodness is the gain of a genuine gratification of graciousness.

My family was faced with a profound choice of deciding whether death is the right to exist with an incurable illness or the right to die with dignity. After my death several organizations criticized my parents for pulling the plug on my life support systems. To them I now say that the choice of becoming one with God is only your family's decision. The fear of finality is a failure of faith. Every day should be a good day to die.

The reality of finality is that each man should be a master of his own death, and a doctor should always help him die without fear of failure or pain. To impose suffering on an unserviceable shell and stopping the spirit of a terminally ill patient from being reborn into the cosmic consciousness is a crime against compassion. Every one of us has a right to a peaceful and dignified death. Only your soul and your family's spirit should decide when it is time to go back to God, and not a statesman.

In our cosmos life and death coexist…and life is of the smaller scale by far. Since people started procreating, over 150 billion of us have been born, but only 6 billion or so of us are still alive. More than 100 million of mankind dies each year.

For longer than the memory of mankind the dead have vastly outnumbered the living. The land of living is limited to years. Only the dead are immortal and immune to illnesses and survive without pain.

With the passing of the physical flesh begins the immortality of your spirit and soul. Physical and psychic energy can only be transformed, not destroyed. Death's essence stretches far from the mortality of your muscles and mind.

Learn to trust your innermost thoughts. The time to change your life is before not knowing just how good living is, and then you find yourself lying cold in your grave. The curable may seek and speak of God's kindness. The incurable may become as one with God by separating the skin, spirit, and soul into an immortality without illness and thus entering a paradise without pain.

Within my pool of perception my mind was now a molecule surrounded by millions of others, and with each contact of another atom of intelligence I gained more knowledge. I now became the proof that energy cannot be destroyed, it only changes shape. When your skin expires your life force energy only changes in form, not functionality.

When you reach out and rise above your doubt and despair they disappear, and in their place appears the difference between what is said is right and what right really should be.

So go with the grace of God or pay the devil his due. What do you have to lose? As diverse as people are, there is an absolute that connects all humans to one another. We will all die. The same as plants sprout, grow, flower, fruit and send forth seeds for regrowth, during our life cycles our souls also seek rebirth and maintain the memory of what they were and what they wish to be. Life and death are not separate experiences. If we wish to die well…we must wish to live well.

Your greatest strength may come from what you have lost, from what you want, or from what you wish for but not yet have. Some days it is only from what you live for. So meanwhile enjoy what you are, as well as what you never want to be. Even an illness can be a great inspiration to improve your life.

So, get over it…get on with it…work through your problems and turn them into opportunities. End the gap between knowing what to do and doing it. Get real! Remember that change is the only constant in this universe.

Become more than a beast to burdens and desires. In all stages of life and death there are moments of opportunity to evolve as a human being. Not all people are destined to do great things while they are living, but all of us can dare to be great at the time of our deaths. By giving life to others, we can help ourselves reach an everlasting eternity.

When you know that death is imminent it can be painful for those who are unprepared and become a terrifying experience. The loss of control of one's life can be devastating. Although death still can even be painful for those who are prepared, being unprepared for your ultimate reality seems such a waste. To ignore and fear what is a natural part of life…is to live an unexamined life. Life and death will always be partners. Since all that blossoms must die, why not leave behind the gift of life and strive to live a life filled with wonderment. Then you can work towards a peaceful evolution of experiencing why our souls are dwelling in the land of the living and not yet joined in the illumination of becoming as one with the *"we in thee"*.

Death can catch us unaware at any time and has no compassion.

Normally when we hear of someone else's death we tend to think it was their turn to die, and of course our turn will never come. But no one escapes life alive. Death always claims its due.

Learn to live the life you imagined. You cannot buy your good health back. To defeat death you must want to live life every day to the fullest. Sadly, too often today only the elderly and terminally ill realize their health is their greatest wealth.

Live your life as if each precious minute is your last. Learn to challenge the core of your existence, and after learning to be as one with the stars, sun, sky and sea, you will attain an intimate contact inside the celestial section of your cranium.

While you seek truer thoughts, sights, sounds, smell, taste and touch, the supreme synergy of spirit, soul and skin you gain will insure that your brain and body will be in the best of balance. Then the sanest sounds you will hear will be the healthful powers of your head, heart and hands working together in holy harmony.

It doesn't get much better when you exceed your expectations and then start on a timeless travel towards the theo-synergy of the wellness of the "*we in thee*". Learn to embrace the flickering flame of fate that faces all of our future fates. Become a soul mate to someone suffering. Learn to laugh out loud, tell the truth and make your word your worldly worth. When you give the gift of life, then your third transcendental eye will open to the timeless thoughts that will turn any tragedy into tranquility.

Some of this writing may seem foolish or over factual. However, when you die young, your humor and huzzah still lives on. When you find yourself speaking from beyond the land of time, you do tend to sound like a teenager trivializing transcendentalism and theosophy. So please forgive my story rambling on and on and on. I died too young to know all the proper rules of recording my remembrances.

Although "the day I died" sounds like the end to a story, in actuality it is about a new beginning. You now know my dying breath beget new beginnings for ten other beings. This story is really about life and death, but at this precise moment it has become difficult to tell them apart. But faith and fact don't have to be opposites…you can't see air, but yet you still know it is there. If you dare accept that this tale may be true, those of faith will now know the secrets of the grave can be yours to explore.

THE DAY I DIED

So now my story has ended, but please indulge a dead boy a few questions for you. What if you or a loved one was dying today, but knew you could be saved...

How far would you go?

How much would you spend?

How long would you wait?

What wouldn't you do to survive?

So become a hero and help save someone in harm's way. Be brave and make the righteous choice to become an organ donor. As our Lord so said, *"Do unto others as you would have them do unto you"*.

Printed in the United States
43349LVS00005B/88-99